Juliana de Lima Soares
Laura Filomena Santos de Araújo
Roseney Bellato

Re-significations and perspectives of the lived

Juliana de Lima Soares
Laura Filomena Santos de Araújo
Roseney Bellato

Re-significations and perspectives of the lived

Experiência de cuidado cotidiano ao filho com a rara Síndrome de Schinzel-Giedion

ScienciaScripts

Imprint

Cover image: www.ingimage.com

This book is a translation from the original published under ISBN 978-3-330-76293-0.

Publisher:
Sciencia Scripts
is a trademark of
Dodo Books Indian Ocean Ltd. and OmniScriptum S.R.L publishing group

120 High Road, East Finchley, London, N2 9ED, United Kingdom
Str. Armeneasca 28/1, office 1, Chisinau MD-2012, Republic of Moldova, Europe
Managing Directors: Ieva Konstantinova, Victoria Ursu
info@omniscriptum.com

Printed at: see last page
ISBN: 978-620-8-38961-1

Dedication

To Jéssica, Bruno and Ricardo.
Thank you for the kind and affectionate way in which you have shared your lives with me. You have become very special to me!

ACKNOWLEDGEMENTS

To God:

To the only one who is worthy to receive honour and glory, to the master of masters, to the lord of lords, I thank you for the countless blessings you have bestowed on me throughout these twenty-five years of life.
To the family:

To my son, Luiz César, who didn't exist in this world at the time this work was being written, but is now the reason for my life. Thank you for making me realise the love I received from my parents. I love you, son!

To my husband, César Androlage, my encourager and companion throughout these eleven years. Thank you for worrying about my future, which is also yours. I love you, love!

To my mum, Roseli, who, with her "roselizinha" way of being, cheers me on, rejoices in my joys and loves me unconditionally. Thank you for all this love without measure. I love you, Mum!

To my father, Hebert Luiz, who, although he was taken from me at a young age, I know that wherever he is, he cheers on my achievements. I love you, Dad!

To my brother, Hebert Junior, thank you for always being by my side, supporting me and cheering on my achievements. I love you, Ju!

To my grandparents, Dina and Faustino, who are two precious jewels for me, as much parents as I am. Thank you for all the valuable teachings you give me every day. I love you, Mum! I love you, Grandad!

To my uncle, Rosevaldo, who with his playful way always advises me and worries about my future. I love you, Uncle!

To my kittens, Lindona, Oncinha, Titã and Avelã, who in times of sadness always give me "purrs" that calm my heart. I love you all!

To my dear friends:

Ítala, for all the times we've laughed and mourned together. Thank you for the privilege of having you by my side from graduation to now. Regardless of the paths we take, I know that our friendship will remain strong... Maybe towards the Dr, right?

Robson, for all the advice and all the moments of joy we shared. Thank you for being a loyal friend and always willing to help. May our friendship continue to walk this flowery and joyful path.

Jonatan, for all your tenderness and friendship over so long. For me, you are synonymous with kindness and love of neighbour.

Hugo, for all the moments of joy that we have shared so far and that we will continue to share. For me, you are synonymous with perseverance and victory.

To the Nursing, Health and Citizenship Research Group:

To my dear and beloved "Profs" Laura and Roseney, who, beyond scientific knowledge, taught me about the essence of the human.

To all the scientific initiation students, masters, master's and doctoral students who have passed through me over these seven years in the "Gepesquiana" family.

Then, suddenly, I experienced "satori": my eyes were opened and I saw as I had never seen before. I realised that time is just a thread. All the experiences of beauty and love that we go through are threaded through it. "What memory has loved remains eternal". A sunset, a letter we receive from a friend, fields of fat grass shining in the rising sun, the scent of jasmine, a single glance from a loved one, soup bubbling on the wood cooker, autumn trees, bathing in a waterfall, hands holding each other, a child's embrace: there have been many moments of such beauty in my life that I've said to myself: "It was worth living my whole life just to be able to experience this moment". There are ephemeral moments that *justify a lifetime.*

I suddenly realised that the pain of the interrupted sonata is due to the fact that we live under the spell of time. We think that life is a sonata that begins with birth and must end with old age. But that's wrong.

We live in time, it's true. But it's eternity that gives life meaning. Eternity is not endless time. Endless time is unbearable. Can you imagine endless music, endless kisses, endless books? Everything beautiful must come to an end. Everything beautiful must die. Beauty and death always go hand in hand.

Eternity is complete time, that time when you say: "It was worth it". There's no need for evolution, no need for transformation. Time is complete and happiness is total. Of course, as Guimarães Rosa says, this only happens in rare moments of distraction. But it doesn't matter. If it happened, it's eternal. As opposed to the "never again" of chronological time, this moment is destined for "forever and ever".

I then realised that life is not a sonata that, in order to achieve its beauty, has to be played to the end. On the contrary, I realised that life is an album of mini-sonatas. Every moment of beauty lived and loved, however ephemeral, is a complete experience that is destined for eternity. A single moment of beauty and love justifies a lifetime.

Fbemm Alves (1999) in the book Concerto para corpo e alma.

SUMMARY

In this book, we cover the experience of a family whose son was born with a very rare syndrome called Schinzel-Giedion (SSG), which is congenital, neurodegenerative and has a bleak prognosis. Our aim was to understand the family's experience of caring for a chronically ill child with a rare syndrome. This is a comprehensive approach in which, assuming that people experience life events in a very personal way, we opted for a "situation study". The participating family is made up of Bruno and Jéssica, a young couple, parents of Ricardo, a one-year-old baby. The methodological strategies included Life History operationalised by In-Depth Interview and Observation. The information was collected between June 2015 and January 2016, and the empirical material was organised in the Research Diary, making up our corpus of analysis. We carried out an attentive reading, highlighting the axes of meaning of the family experience: a) caring in the situation of a rare illness: the family's experience and the resolving capacity of the health services and b) the resignifications and perspectives of the experience of having a child with the rare Schinzel-Giedion Syndrome. The matrix research to which this study is linked has ethical approval No. 951.101/CEP-HUJM/2015. Aware of the short life expectancy imposed by SSG, the family is extremely active, travelling beyond the geographical limits of the state where they live in an attempt to obtain some help in providing the best care for their child. The element of 'time' is particularly important, since it is in time that Ricardo's life takes place and it is also in time that he suffers the uncertain tomorrows imposed by the very rare SSG. The family makes the most of this time in their son's life, both in terms of extending it as much as possible and offering the best care "of, in and for" life. Jéssica and Bruno's expectations in relation to parenthood have been re-signified over time, and the young couple continue to learn how to be a family within Ricardo's possible normality, taking care of the needs inherent to a baby and also those imposed by the SSG. They continue to live 'with' and 'for' their son, intensely enjoying the "here and now" in order to expand the present, with the becoming constituted by the projection of what is lived. Finally, we grasp the notion of care that encompasses and integrates the needs of the beginning of human life, flowing and spreading to care during illness, for which promptness and speed are essential. It encourages us to think about the concept of time as a confluence in which past and future overlap the present, which is an inexhaustible source of the lived, through which life flows ceaselessly. Health services and professionals need to consider the different notions of time and temporality, rethinking the protocol and rigidly formalised times that, as a rule, guide their actions and the organisation of care processes, in an effort to embrace the temporality of living and caring for children with other normalities.

SUMMARY

CHAPTER 1 7

CHAPTER 2 11

CHAPTER 3 12

CHAPTER 4 16

CHAPTER 5 26

CHAPTER 6 34

CHAPTER 7 45

CHAPTER 8 51

CHAPTER 1

INTRODUCTION

This study is part of the matrix research "Subsidies for Modelling the Care of Families in Situations of Vulnerability", the aim of which is to understand the potential of families in situations of vulnerability to support the modelling of care, and is the responsibility of the Nursing Health and Citizenship Research Group (GPESC).

The GPESC has developed research from the privileged perspective of people and their families, taking an interest in the family experience of care, with an emphasis on living through the chronic situation of illness and, in this living, the provision and management of care for life and health (BELLATO, 2011).

I joined the Group in 2009, when I was part of the matrix research project "The legal institution as a mediator in the realisation of the national right to health: analysis of therapeutic itineraries of users/families in the SUS/MT" (DITSUS), and, as a scientific initiation scholarship holder, my study aimed to analyse court decisions involving demands for surgeries in the Mato Grosso Court of Justice (TJMT) when the state denied the demand. This study brought me closer to the theme of chronic illness, as a large part of the court cases involved the multiple care needs it entails, contrasting with what is strictly legally demanded and punctually guaranteed by the health field; as well as the family experience of care in this situation. In this way, I observed that "[...] the effectiveness of the right to health, provided by the mediation of the TJMT, occurred only with regard to a strictly cut-out need" (SOARES et al., 2011, p.899), greatly affecting the experience of family care.

This first experience initiated me into scientific research and, since then, I have been developing studies involving family care in chronic illness situations.

In a second step, I covered the care-seeking trajectory of an elderly woman with a chronic condition and her family in order to understand the different ways in which bonds are woven into the healthcare sphere, with an emphasis on the bond woven by the person and the one established by the healthcare professional (SOARES et al., 2013a). Thus, this study also brought me closer to the notion of longitudinality in healthcare, precepted by Starfield (2002, p.247) "as a long-term personal relationship between health professionals and patients in their health units", which is fundamental in chronic care, since it enables professionals to get to know people, considering their values and needs, in order to be a reference for care for the person and their family.

On the other hand, the Nursing Degree Final Paper allowed me to shed light on the weaving of the bond in the professional relationship between the sick person and the family in a chronic illness situation, demonstrating it as an important element in guaranteeing the longitudinal care that such a situation requires, with the professional being responsible for weaving it into the relationship with the family (SOARES et al., 2013b).

These studies have had repercussions on my academic practice since graduation, awakening my gaze to the importance of considering the multiple dimensions of human life, even in a one-off care situation in a hospital environment. I gradually realised the immense responsibility involved in caring for a human being who, like me, carries their own values and feelings that are not abdicated when they are ill and, therefore, must be taken into account by health professionals.

In this way, immersing myself in the scientific and academic practice of family care has made me aware of the immense value that the family has in people's lives, as well as realising the countless and meticulous care that it provides for each of its loved ones and for the multiple dimensions of living, including the onset of illness. So, eager to pursue my academic career, I entered the Master's programme with an interest in studying topics related to the family care experience.

In order to understand this experience, it is necessary to enter the world of the family, in an effort to get closer and try to "be part of" their time-place, even if in a circumscribed way and within the scope of a research project.

In studies based on Matrix Research[1] , everyday life is taken to be the world of the lived experience that arouses our research interests, with the "home" being a privileged place where things happen and take on their own meanings that are close to people, inscribed in the rhythms of routine, taking on shapes that are closer to habit than to the chronometer (BELLATO et al., 2011). We therefore emphasise the notion of 'home-nest' presented by Bachelard (1993) as our place of origin, where we return or dream of returning, just as a bird returns to its nest and a lamb returns to its fold.

> This sign of return marks infinite daydreams, because human returns are made on the great rhythm of human life, a rhythm that crosses the years, which fights against all absences through dreams. A component of intimate fidelity resonates in the approximate images of the nest and the house (BACHELARD, 1993, p. 262).

In this sense, the lived world is governed by an experiential temporality, which "shapes the ways in which each person perceives and gives meaning to the time lived in the present, combining it with their past and future anticipations" (DOLINA; BELLATO; ARAÚJO, 2014, p.78).

We corroborate the idea that "[...] the reality of experiential time is at odds with the time of cold hours - the physical time that is independent of us" (BELLATO; ARAÚJO, 2015). As such, the extension and expansion of lived time, beyond the counting of the hours, takes place through the subjective apprehension of the duration of events (BACHELARD, 1994).

In our approach to the experience of illness, we are therefore interested in this non-linear time, known as "experiential temporality", which was approached by the research group through the study by Dolina, Bellato and Araújo (2014, p.82), which aimed to understand the reflections and contrasts between experiential temporality and the time of protocol therapy, in the experience of a young woman with breast cancer. In it, the authors point out that "the logic of what is experienced, in the simultaneity of events that mobilise the intense suffering that cancer produces, deforms and reshapes time in another dimension, which is certainly not linear".

Thus, we presuppose that each family member has their own very personal "way of life"; and that, in

---

[1] Subsidies for modelling care for families in situations of vulnerability developed by the Nursing, Health and Citizenship Research Group at the Federal University of Mato Grosso.

everyday family life, the affective-relational time-place, the "ways of life" formed in the relationship between the different members mould their own ways of "being and caring as a family". In this sense, we highlight the home as the place where these complex family relationships take place, which gives it an affective reference beyond the possession of a physical space, making it an essential requirement for family life (PORTUGAL, 2014).

This makes us confident that our research endeavours are an approximate attempt to get to know the family care experience based on what the people themselves can tell us about this experience, which is individual at the same time as it is lived collectively. It is therefore necessary to cultivate sensitivity in order to perceive how situations are experienced by them, as they gradually shape their ways of being and acting, in a confluence between being-living and living-being. In this way, we understand that what we are has an intense and particular relationship with our ways of living, and the reciprocal is also possible.

In this context, it must be understood that if each situation is unique and personal, so is the situation of chronic illness. And this brief account of our trajectory lends coherence to the choice of theme for this study, in which we cover the experience of a family whose son was born with a rare syndrome, called Schinzel-Giedion (SSG), which is congenital, neurodegenerative and has a bleak prognosis, with death in the first few years of life. The participating family is made up of Bruno and Jéssica, a young couple aged 23 and 24 respectively, parents of Ricardo, who was born in June 2014 and was one year old at the time of this study.

SSG was first described in 1978 by two researchers, Albert Schinzel and Andreas Giedion, and is characterised by an autosomal dominant genetic disorder (HOISCHEN et al., 2010) that causes numerous health problems for newborns.

In Brazil, there are few studies on the syndrome, and research by Albano et al. (2004), with the aim of highlighting bilateral congenital hydronephrosis in the diagnosis of GHS, described the first Brazilian case of a newborn with this syndrome. At the time, Albano et al. (2004) listed 35 cases described in the literature. A more recent study, which described the first case of a child with SGA in Spain, points out that only 52 cases have been reported worldwide so far (GONZÁLES et al., 2015). A study by Carvalho et al. (2015) is the most recent to describe two clinical cases in Brazilian children.

According to the family taking part in this study, in an intensive search they carried out, they learnt of three confirmed cases in Brazil, of which only their baby, Ricardo, is still alive. As such, this study endeavours to cover a particularly unique situation, full of meticulous care for Ricardo's life.

We should also emphasise that health care for families who experience any kind of illness is already a challenging task, especially given the multiplicity and complexity of the elements involved in providing care, with an emphasis on the specific contexts of life and health, as well as the effectiveness of formal care systems in modifying people's health situation (GERHARDT et al., 2010).

We would point out that this challenge is greatly intensified when it comes to a rare illness since, in addition to all the difficulties faced by services in meeting the multiple needs demanded by people and their families, its rarity brings with it specificities that require specialised professional attention. There is still little solidified knowledge about these diseases, which delays the time it takes to make a diagnosis, as well as hindering the therapy needed to care for these people. It is therefore necessary to reflect on the need for professional practices to be modelled on family care, supporting it in its own right (BELLATO et al., 2016).

This justifies the effort to understand the specificities of the very peculiar situation of illness resulting from HGS, which entails countless compromises for the life of the child and their family, including death as a near possibility, in order to offer support to services and professionals so that they can support families in their needs and expand the potential intrinsic to them.

With this understanding, I will present the family in this study in such a way as to give personalisation and life to discussions that start from the concrete reality of people's ways of living, and are therefore simultaneously singular and universal, since lived experiences carry with them transcendence and the possibility of recognition between human beings (BELLATO; ARAÚJO, 2015).

CHAPTER 2

GENERAL OBJECTIVE

To understand the family's experience of day-to-day care while living with a rare, compromising syndrome that limits their child's life in their early years.

CHAPTER 3

INTRODUCING RICARDO'S FAMILY

It is worth emphasising that instead of assuming a concept of what a family is - in terms of its structure and/or conformation - we have chosen to "flesh out" the family in this study in order to make visible the family's own experience of care in a situation. Thus, we have in mind that in order to get to know a family, as well as knowing how to listen, you need to be sensitive enough to see between the lines and grasp what it carries implicitly within itself (OLIVEIRA; MARCON, 2007).

As this is a 'newly enlarged' family that is organised around and as a result of its first child, we decided to name it after the child, given its centrality in the parents' attention and care. In this way, I present the drawing of the Genogram covering three generations of Ricardo's Family, with an emphasis on the nucleus of care, made up of him, the one-year-old baby and his parents, Bruno and Jéssica. The drawing is accompanied by excerpts from observations and narratives that also highlight the family experience.

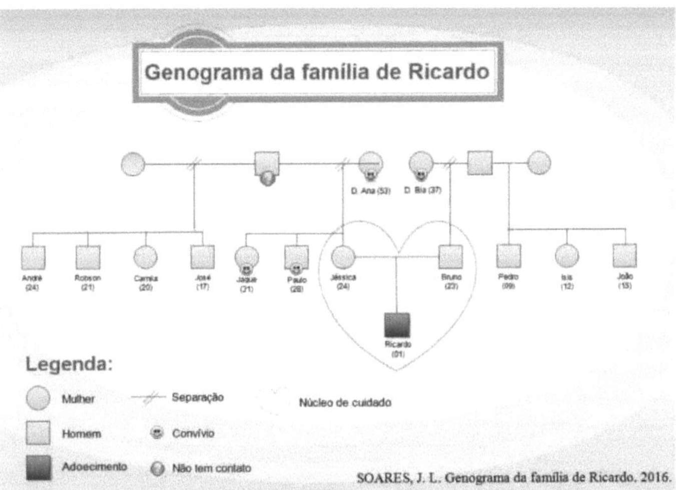

Figure 1 - Genogram of Ricardo's family

Jéssica and Bruno started dating when they were sixteen and got married when they were eighteen. Six years later, they decided to have a baby and started planning for Jéssica to become pregnant, but Ricardo came along sooner than expected:

> It was like that, we always said that when I finished university, right? And we already had the house, we were practically ready to hand it over [...] because I wanted to, even in my last... a month before I knew I was pregnant, I'd had my check-up with the gynaecologist. I even spoke to my gynaecologist and said: "Next year I want to get pregnant", right? I told him, like, Ricardo came six months before my due date, right? But it was kind of planned (Jéssica, mum).

Throughout the thirty-six weeks of pregnancy and as they attended prenatal appointments, the couple received occasional information about the possibility of their baby being born with some alterations, but the surprise came when Jéssica gave birth: We knew about a few problems during the pregnancy, but nothing like this. Then when he was born, he was born with a lot of things!" (Bruno, father)

Thus, after his birth and because of his prematurity, as well as the health problems caused by the syndrome, it was necessary for Ricardo to remain in the Neonatal Intensive Care Unit (NICU) for the first month of his life:

> And until then he stayed in the ICU, he was in the ICU for a month and a bit, right? he had tests and stuff... and... in the ICU, there's a test that's done which is the karyotype, which looks at the DNA and so on, to see if there's any syndrome or not... And his was normal! And then, when he came out, he had the ear test, the foot test... Everything was altered, except the foot test (Bruno, father).
>
> [...] I only remember that in the late afternoon, when I wanted to see him [Ricardo] because I didn't really remember him, when he was born... then I couldn't because I couldn't even stand up, so... and even if I could stand up, I had to have had a bath to get into the neonatal ICU. So I couldn't see him the first day he was born. Then on the second day, when I went to... on the day he was discharged, I had a bath and went to see him... but he was so tiny, this little baby [tunes her voice to speak in a very affectionate way]... (Jéssica, mum)

Ricardo is the couple's first child and, as such, was eagerly awaited by his parents. Although he is very small for his age, the syndrome he experiences is not so visible at first glance:

> At a glance, he seemed to me to be a baby like all the others, but when I looked more closely I noticed that his forehead was a little wider and his eyes were more "droopy". I then did some research and discovered that these are some of the characteristic signs of the syndrome. Ricardo was also wearing a small gastrostomy tube, but I only noticed it after a while. When we arrived, he was crying a lot and seemed irritable. As time went by and he was cuddled by his mum, he became calmer and even slept *on her lap for a* while (Observation notes - 11.06.2015).

After thirty-four days, two operations and many tests, Ricardo was finally discharged from the NICU and the couple were able to take their son home. However, they carried with them many uncertainties and anxieties, because they knew that their son might have a rare syndrome, but they didn't have a diagnosis.

> *Then... we came out of the ICU, a lot of doctors started... Wow, we went to 10 or 12 doctors... You know... I stopped my life, her life* [referring to Jéssica] *and I ran around every day. Every day, check-ups, check-ups. And then his little problems started appearing... and then we started adapting. That's when we started seeing a geneticist...* [...] *we went there and had our appointments and so on, and a month later... he called us there, right? When we got there, he opened the book he'd studied, researched a lot, was writing in... the book was all in English. He said: oh... everything he has fits this syndrome, but... We're going to do some tests and stuff and...* [...] *until then we knew that he had it, that he wasn't normal, he had a few problems, we didn't know what, right?* [...] *Then... at the weekend, on Friday, he started having these spasms... and we thought it was a break. It was all: Oh, it's a break, it's a break... Well, it would have been, wouldn't it? Then we got there and started to get a bit bigger, then we got there and went to tell him* [the geneticist] *about it. He said: Ah, the first thing that appears in the syndrome here is CONVULSION!* [...] *Then he went to research where the syndrome was tested, right? There were only three laboratories in São Paulo... and we did some research...* [...] *Ninety days to send the results of the test...* (Bruno, father)

Ricardo was born with the rare SSG and this condition imposed several changes on the couple's life, forcing them to readjust their expectations regarding the care of their first child.

So the couple set up an *online* page where they tell us a little about how they found out that their son wasn't going to be born according to their expectations:

> How it all began
> At 5 months gestation, during the morphological ultrasound, we received our first news. My umbilical cord had a peculiarity called AUU (Single Umbilical Artery), and soon afterwards a malformation was seen in Ricardo's hands, called Polydactyly. Until then everything was fine, but the biggest concern came when the doctor told us that there was another problem: Ricardo could have kidney cysts, which would be another malformation that could characterise a syndrome, which could be mild or not. Thus, following the pregnancy closely, a hypertrophy of the right ventricle of the heart was found, which was ruled out by more specialised tests. At 36 weeks gestation, the placenta was no longer sending nutrients to Ricardo, so I went into labour and Ricardo was born prematurely at 7am at the hospital. [...] At birth, we received further news from Ricardo's paediatrician that he had a genital malformation, which was later diagnosed as peno-scrotal hypospadias. Ricardo was immediately taken to the neonatal ICU, where he needed a mechanical respirator for five days, and then HOOD for a further five days. Due to his difficulty in feeding, Ricardo was unable to feed through the breast, which was stimulated for more than a month, and with the difficulties he started feeding with Pre Nan for 45 days. During his hospitalisation, he had a urinary infection, which was treated, and several tests were carried out and assessed by various doctors. Cardiologist: Cystolic murmur in the heart; Dilation of the right chambers; Persistence of a very small arterial canal; Geneticist: Polydactyly in the hands; Hypospadias; Low implantation of the ear; coarse cheeks; complete duplication of the 5th toes. Nephrologist: Bilateral hydronephrosis Pap smear: Normal Eye test: Bilateral Absent Ear test: Altered Transfontanelle ultrasound: Normal Karyotype: Normal (46 XY) Throughout the hospital stay, the most awaited news was this last test, which would determine which syndrome Ricardo would have. The happiness of the normal test was incredible. This happiness only lasted a short time. Continued... "in edition". (Jéssica, mum - extract from *online* page*)*

Jessica's pregnancy and childbirth were periods marked by insecurity and unpredictability in the life of this newly enlarged family, which continues to this day, and the parents have learnt, in everyday life, how to look after their child and the complications that illness imposes on their development.

> [...] *he pooped last night. I usually take it out when I'm bathing him, right? With a tube, I put the little laxative in the syringe, then I put it in the tube, then I put aaa, I put the little tube in the syringe, then I put a little* jhonson® *oil, then I put it in his little bum too, then I go and put it in. But he's very small. Sometimes I prefer to put it in when he's calm, because sometimes it doesn't bother him much* (Jéssica, mum).

Bruno, who is a photographer and cameraman, usually records moments with his son through photographs and videos: And I film him every day, all the time... Every day I film, I take photos... there are more photos of him there... [Continues to show me the photos on his mobile phone] (Bruno, father)

Jéssica has a degree in administration and currently doesn't work in the field, devoting herself exclusively to caring for her family, especially her son:

> Jéssica is like... Jéssica is 24 hours for him now. She doesn't work, she doesn't do anything else. So she... graduated, then got pregnant, then... She was still working, right? And she had a problem in her job too, because the company practically went bankrupt here, but it's based in another city and so on. [...] But since then, she's left the service and had him, right?

The family currently lives in the same neighbourhood as Jéssica's mother and this geographical proximity allows Ricardo to live more closely with his relatives on his mother's side. The couple have shown that they are a nuclear family, although they have many friendships outside of the family's intimacy and also in their own home.

CHAPTER 4

THEORETICAL OUTLINE

The theoretical framework for this study was drawn up on the basis of the research experience itself, in order to support us in understanding the life history of Ricardo's family. Therefore, this outline was built up as the fieldwork developed, giving it its own very personal characteristic, as it was directed by what was experienced and felt by the family, thus forming the substrate for understanding what was specific to them. This openness to the field was made possible by my long immersion in the research group's own theoretical elaboration, in a very close relationship with language and the theoretical-methodological discussions that have taken place within it since my first study plan within it. It certainly constitutes the comprehensive framework on the family experience of care.

So we don't have an "a priori theoretical generality", but a "theoretical context" that allows us to outline the contours of the family's experience (verbal information)[2] . Therefore, the theoretical outline comes from the effort to be impressed by the family's experience, so that the investigation is "embodied in human experience, always local, proper, substantiated, expressing its relevance and meanings" (BELLATO; ARAÚJO, 2015, p. 1396).

Below we present the theoretical outline of this study, which focused on the following themes: a) The family and its potential for care; b) Experiencing a rare chronic illness and the first child with Schinzel-Giedion syndrome; and c) Time and the temporalities of what is experienced.

4.1 The family and its potential for care

> After talking about the diagnosis of the syndrome, Bruno became emotional and, with teary eyes, said that his son's life expectancy was between two and three years, but that they would do anything to give *their son* a good *life* (Observation notes - 11.06.2015, emphasis added).

The family is the pillar of support for the birth, growth and development of its members. This importance is even reflected in the Universal Declaration of Human Rights (1948), right in its preamble, which recognises the inherent dignity of all members of the human family and their equal and inalienable rights as the foundation of freedom, justice and peace in the world.

Such recognition allows us to assimilate a little of the immense value of the family for human society, as it is the place where the first values that people carry with them for life are learnt.

Thus, the family can be conceived as a social body in which a network of relationships and interactions prevails, whose beliefs are manifested in a cultural space (OLIVEIRA; MARCON, 2007). In this way, the family can be thought of as a system that moves through time but, unlike other organisations, its main value is relationships, which are irreplaceable (CARTER; MCGOLDRICK, 2007). Therefore, health care must be understood in the context of the relationships between its members, given the influence of a member's health

---

[2] Roseney Bellato, Cuiabá - MT, 14th September 2015.

on the family group and vice versa (OLIVEIRA; MARCON, 2007).

Thus, the family is a place of mutual support, as the onset of illness not only has repercussions on the life of the person experiencing it, but also on the lives of those directly involved, cared for and afflicted by their suffering (ALMEIDA; ARAÚJO; BELLATO, 2014). In this sense, we start from the premise that the family is the first and main provider of care in all areas of life, including when one or more of their loved ones becomes ill.

Thus, family care is broadly considered by us as care that is essential to life and health, ranging from emotional interactions for a healthy life to learning the habits that contribute to this (GUITIERREZ; MINAYO, 2010). We therefore corroborate the understanding that the family takes care of life and for life in order to provide and/or re-establish the health of their loved ones (BELLATO et al., 2016).

What we are talking about, then, is a notion of care that encompasses and integrates human needs, distancing itself to a large extent from the reductionist cuts proposed by the biomedical view of the sick body. And because it is capable of flowing in different directions, family care spreads throughout people's lives, encompassing their multiple and changing needs over time. As such, care enters the smallest spaces of life, sometimes barely perceptible at first glance, but which occupy a substantially important place in shaping the being.

In this sense, Bellato et al. (2015) talk about the "myriad of care" provided by the family to each of their loved ones throughout their lives. This idea seeks to highlight the abundance of family care, which is subtle, diverse, multiple and barely visible, going beyond what is rationalised as care by the health field (BELLATO et al., 2016). We are therefore interested in making family care visible in its various ways, times and places, assuming that it is integrative and shared within the family. Therefore:

> [...] the experience of care and illness remains integrated into the whole of what is lived, but gains the nuances of a *composé* from the 'tones' given to this experience by each of the family members [...] showing us how each member is affected and affects this family experience (BELLATO; ARAÚJO, 2015, p. 1397).

The onset of illness significantly affects the multiple dimensions of people's daily lives. We are therefore moving away from the idea of illness as a morbid, biological and physical entity, broadening the notion of illness as being part of life, constituting an event that is amalgamated with living itself (BELLATO et al., 2011).

In addition, family care is shared by its various members in a dynamic, plural and changing way, and they exchange different elements of care in the various situations they experience (BELLATO et al., 2016), depending on the conditions they have available to do so.

In this way, the family's care potentials are understood as a set of resources, capacities, means, dispositions, among others, available to or mobilised by people in the daily dimension of life, governing the possibilities for their care to prosper (verbal information) .[3]

Thus, each family member is potency in essence, as Almeida, Araújo and Bellato (2014) found in their

[3] Laura Filomena Santos de Araújo, Research group meeting, Cuiabá - MT, February 2014.

study on family care in a young person's experience of chronic illness. This means that the form of expression of human potency is singular and personalised, so that each person offers what they have, whether in terms of involvement, readiness, attitude and acts of care. The synergy of these powers in constant movement therefore offers a certain support in coping with a situation of illness.

In this way, the potential for care needs to refer to the person themselves, their family and the community they belong to, and it matters to us how, "in situation", the various potentials are transmuted from their latent form into support, help, sustenance and support for care (verbal information) .[4]

The onset of illness requires the family to devise new forms of care, specific to the new situation that is emerging, without giving up those that were already present in life. Thus, each member of the family can mobilise their caring powers, with family care resulting from the diverse potentialities modelled on the situations that arise and the contingencies of what is experienced, so as to enable the best way of dealing with them.

Becoming ill certainly imposes new ways of organising care on the family, causing it to arrange and rearrange itself with the potential it has, be it material, human, affective, relational, among others (MUFATO et al., 2012). In this sense, Souza and Lima (2007) emphasise that illness, especially chronic illness, brings with it the creation of new normalities in people's lives, different from the previous one. These normalities help people to cope with the chronic situation of illness, as they increase their chances of being happy.

When it comes to a newly formed family, there are expectations about the first child and how to look after it. These expectations have been evident for a long time and Fiamenghi Jr and Messa (2007) point out that parents often idealise a child in their minds and so, from the beginning of the pregnancy, they often imagine the baby's sex, think about its school performance, career, sexual orientation, among other expectations.

In the case of young parents, the onset of illness seems to impose "learning to be a family" at the same time as "learning to care while ill", and care relationships are shaped in this context. Thus, we agree that care relationships presuppose weaving and reweaving family ties, in a renewable continuum that shapes family care (MUSQUIM, 2013). We also agree with the authors that living with a chronic illness requires people to be able to deal with the challenges that arise, overcoming them so as not to restrict their way of life to the limitations imposed by this illness (SOUZA; LIMA, 2007).

We emphasise that the potential and support that the family has and engenders allows them, to a certain extent, to deal with situations of vulnerability more or less effectively, making it possible to maintain the necessary care for their various loved ones (BELLATO et al., 2016). Young parents therefore find themselves in a situation where they need to put their powers into action, shaping them to cope with the new circumstances that arise in their lives.

However, if this situation of illness persists over time, the family's potential for care can be exhausted; and this happens more intensely to the extent that these situations have a considerable impact on their concrete possibilities for care. Thus, in their way of living and caring, the family can be vulnerable in different ways

---

[4] Laura Filomena Santos de Araújo, Research group meeting, Cuiabá - MT, February 2014.

and express it in different ways, which can be extended as a result of the lack of sustainability of family care on the part of health services and professionals (BELLATO et al, 2016).

In this way, we consider that the family is not "vulnerable" a priori, but can "find itself" in situations of vulnerability. Therefore, vulnerability must be contextualised as a situation, because it "conjugates in the plural", and is not a fixed situation, nor is it permanent or of a single nature (BELLATO et al, 2016).

We note that the issue of vulnerability has been discussed by the scientific community as an innovative and important proposal in the field of public health (AYRES et al., 2003; SÁNCHEZ, BERTOLOZZI, 2007; OVIEDO, CZERESNIA, 2014). For our part, we are interested in the perspective of families in situations of vulnerability and how they deal with these situations.

By understanding the care potentials mobilised by people and their families, as well as their ways of caring and being cared for, we aim to provide support so that health professionals, especially nurses, can offer protective practices to families in order to strengthen them in their care potentials, supporting them in coping with situations of vulnerability (UNIVERSIDADE FEDERAL DE MATO GROSSO, 2014).

Based on this discussion of family care in the context of chronic illness, we believe it is important to contextualise it, now with regard to the specific characteristics of illness, which, as well as being chronic, carries the specificity of syndromic rarity and a gloomy prognosis. We would like to point out that the vast majority of studies on rare diseases take a clinical approach and are based on case studies of the disease. We therefore believe that this research makes a major contribution to the literature, as it was developed from the perspective of the family experiencing the rare illness and brings humanity to a panorama that has been discussed in the clinical and diagnostic spheres.

4.2 Experiencing a rare chronic illness: the only child with Schinzel-Giedion syndrome

> Ricardo began to cry a lot. Jessica calmly tried to find out what was happening to her son, applied some medicine to his nose because he had the flu and a runny nose, but he continued to cry. She then turned him face down on his legs, so that his weight was on his stomach. She told us that when he has colic, this is the best position, and she was right, it was colic. He gradually calmed down and even laid his head on *her palm.* (Observation notes - 02.07.2015)

The birth of their first child is an important moment in the life of the couple, who gradually begin to shift the centre of their attention from their relationship as a couple to the child they will have. Thus, it is from the first child that the new family is formed. McGoldrick (2007) talks about this transition, emphasising that with the birth of the first child, the family becomes a group of three people, forming a permanent system that survives even if one of the people leaves the triad. Thus, with the birth of a child, the family will never break up, even if there is the possibility of separation or even the death of one of the spouses, the family body will continue to exist made up of those who still make it up.

The change to this stage of life requires the couple to move up a generation in the family, now becoming adult carers for a younger generation (CARTER; MCGOLDRICK, 2007). This transition in the family life cycle is felt by the parents in various spheres of daily life, as they begin to organise themselves for the baby's first care (FIAMENGHI JR.; MESSA, 2007).

Thus, immersed in feelings and expectations, the couple is expecting their first child. However, the news that their child will be born with a congenital disorder requires the parents to readjust to the new scenario, changing their plans and expectations.

And if illness is relevant when it takes place chronically, often gradually and over a long period of time, how can we assess the effects on the family when it starts abruptly, even during the intrauterine formation of the new being, who will come into the world already in a situation of illness that will last for years to come? Faced with this, the family continues to modify daily life to accommodate their demands, singularities, modulations and reliefs in order to re-signify the experience of parenthood and future life plans "for" and "with" the child.

Understanding this other way of installing chronicity and the ways in which it affects life is necessary if we are to grasp it in its living thickness, since it is experienced by people and expressed in various dimensions - through suffering, gestures, attitudes, terms, complaints (BELLATO et al., 2011).

In the field of health care, the understanding that a disease can present itself in a more or less persistent form has called into question the traditional division between communicable diseases and chronic non-communicable diseases, given that certain communicable diseases, due to the long period of their natural course, would be closer to the logic of dealing with chronic diseases. This led to a new understanding of health problems as "acute conditions" or "chronic conditions" (MENDES, 2012).

Acute conditions are those that start suddenly, are short-lived and respond well to specific treatments; chronic conditions, on the other hand, are those that start and evolve slowly, usually with multiple causes that vary over time (MENDES, 2012). These conditions have in common the fact that they persist and require a certain level of permanent care (WHO, 2002).

Thus, the World Health Organisation (WHO) defines chronic conditions as health problems that require continuous management by people and health services over a period of several years or decades (WHO, 2002).

A person and their family's experience of a chronic condition is characterised by the fact that it is not temporary, since it becomes part of their lives, either for a prolonged period or for an indefinite period (SOUZA, 2006). As such, we consider the length of time for which the chronic condition lasts to be fundamental, and it can even become a permanent condition, as is the case with the syndrome focussed on in this study.

In addition, in order to broaden the WHO definition of chronic condition, which is still focussed on the disease, we have taken the concept of chronic situation proposed by Bellato et al. (2016) as one that involves becoming ill and the many types of care required, as well as the various effects of becoming ill and the search for care on the lives of the sick person and their family.

Thus, the understanding of the chronic situation presented here seeks to broaden the view of the multiple contingencies that weigh on people and their families when they experience illness and, in it, the concrete possibilities for them to take care of themselves and be taken care of, highlighting the modes of existence that sustain their care (BELLATO et al., 2016), this considered in relation to the time they live in.

We would emphasise that in a chronic situation due to congenital illness, there is an intense confluence of becoming ill and living, since the baby is already born ill and this is the "normality" possible in their life. This situation also has repercussions on the parents, who shape their way of living and caring, taking into account the needs inherent in their child's stage of life and those demanded by the illness.

Thus, these elements are related to the family's time in life, since if, on the one hand, being "born" with compromises and limitations in life leads to various re-significations by the parents in relation to their child, on the other hand, the onset of an illness that limits the child's time in life, permanently compromising it in its first few years, greatly emphasises the need for parents to learn to deal with this situation.

In this sense, Souza (2006) states that there are various "normalities" present in the different ways of going through life, making them flexible, dynamic and changeable. Thus, parents are potentially the best indicators of intervention paths that health professionals can follow (SILVA; BELLATO; ARAÚJO, 2013), since they are the ones who know their ways of going through life.

In addition, the rarity of a congenital syndrome such as the one covered in this study also has repercussions on the possibilities of caring for the child. Scientific studies that could support professional health practices are very limited, which makes it very difficult to provide care in this situation, in terms of medical diagnosis, treatment, maintenance of care over time, among other things.

Ordinance No. 199 of 30 January 2014, which establishes the National Policy for Comprehensive Care for People with Rare Diseases, defines in its article 3 that "a rare disease is one that affects up to 65 people per 100,000 individuals, i.e. 1.3 people per 2,000 individuals" (BRASIL, 2014, p.3).

It's worth noting that for most of these illnesses there are no specific drugs, only supportive treatment such as physiotherapy and speech therapy (FIOVARANTI, 2014).

The São Paulo State Research Foundation (FAPESP) released a report on the distribution of genetic disorders in the country, showing that in Brazil it is estimated that around 13 million people have a rare disease, and that around the world 6,000 different types have been described, most of them of genetic origin (FIOVARANTI, 2014).

Orphanet, the reference portal for information on rare diseases and orphan drugs[5] , published the Rare Disease Prevalence Report in May 2014, highlighting the difficulty of knowing the prevalence of a rare disease:

> "There is a low level of consistency between studies, poor documentation of the methods used, confusion between incidence and prevalence, and/or confusion between incidence at birth and incidence throughout life" (p. 2).

As already mentioned, care for rare diseases in Brazil is provided for in the National Policy for Comprehensive Care for People with Rare Diseases, which has the following objectives:

---

[5] So-called "orphan" drugs are those aimed at treating diseases that are so rare that there is a reluctance to develop them under normal commercialisation conditions, as the small market does not allow the capital invested in the research and development of the product to be recovered. In order to stimulate research and development in the orphan drug sector, public authorities implement incentives for the health and biotechnology industries. An example of this is the adoption of the Orphan Drug Act in 1983 in the United States.

> [...] "reduce mortality, contribute to the reduction of morbidity and mortality and secondary manifestations and improve people's quality of life, through promotion, prevention, early detection, timely treatment, disability reduction and palliative care" (BRASIL, 2014, p.3).

This policy distributes responsibilities to the various state bodies, ranging from guaranteeing health services and human resources in the field of diseases, with the qualification of professionals to work in the area, to monitoring, evaluation and auditing mechanisms, with a view to improving the quality of actions (BRASIL, 2014).

With specific regard to SSG, González et al. (2014) emphasise its severity and lethality, describing that the majority of children affected by the syndrome die in the first few years of life due to mutations in the SETBP1 gene. This gene was mapped by Hoischen et al. (2010) and its mutation would be responsible for the severity of the disease's symptoms, which include genital and renal anomalies, seizures, growth deficiency and severe mental disability, among others.

Lehman et al. (2008) suggest that the clinical diagnosis can be made by identifying facial features - which include frontal hump, midface retraction, anteverted nostrils, hypertrichosis, among others - plus at least one of the two main distinguishing features: bone anomalies or hydronephrosis.

Furthermore, the karyotype test is not capable of diagnosing SSG, and a specific partial sequencing test of one of the segments of the mutated gene - exon 4 of SETBP1 - is required to confirm the syndrome (CARVALHO et al., 2015).

Thus, we understand that there are still challenges to be overcome, such as facilitating children's access to available treatments and supplies, as well as the need for greater organisation of the health network and the social and family support network (MARTINS et al., 2012).

As the condition is congenital, permanent and rare, it imposes an unexpected situation on the parents when it comes to caring for their new family member. In this way, they have to make an intense effort to find support from different sources and places to help them provide the best care for their child. The seriousness of the illness and the knowledge of its lethality can lead to a cascade of feelings about their child and the uncertainty of tomorrow.

Thus, the permanence of the illness in the family's life implies various re-significations of the ways of living and caring, causing them to change their future plans "for" and "with" the child. We therefore consider it relevant to present, in the following topic, a discussion on the different temporalities of family life in order to get closer to the notions of time and its repercussions on living with and caring for a child whose future is cut short by congenital illness.

4.3 Time and the temporality of the lived

> At the end of the visit, after we had switched off the recorders, Jessica gave us some beautiful words about her relationship with her son and the way she faces this "tight" time of life. She said that she prefers to enjoy today, day after day, and that the important thing is that right now she has her son in her arms, making it clear that the future is something you can't control (Observation notes - 02.07.2015, emphasis added).

We know that lived situations take place in time, but what is this time?
Such an enquiry gives rise to a multitude of possible answers and, in general, we would say that time is the whole of what 'happened', what 'is happening' and what 'will happen'; and that it follows the division "past, present and future" whose meanings cover the many human experiences, forming part of the human being and their deepest expectations.

We must emphasise that the perception of time is not univocal or perennial, undergoing important changes throughout human history. Thompson (1998) points out the fundamental contrast between the times of nature and those established by the industrial revolution. For the author, it is true that the rooster has an immemorial role as nature's clock, in a time that is cyclical; the clock mechanism, on the other hand, transforms the perception of time for modern people, as chronological time, an image that expands for many reasons "[...] until, with Newton, it takes over the universe" (THOMPSON, 1998, p.269).

Because we are heirs to this tradition, the "chronologisation" of time in seconds, minutes, hours, days, weeks, months, years etc. is part of our everyday landscape. And the profusion of resources for observing it shows the preponderance of the linear understanding of time that chronologically marks the organising processes of a large part of social life. Thus, our different activities each follow a certain chronological time, forming "overlapping layers" or "temporal extracts", because there must be a time to study, to work, to rest, to produce, to plant, among other human activities.

This preponderance of chronological time seems to subterranean another essential presence in human life, the sense of which is expressed as "temporality" because it is a subjectively perceived, experiential time. Let's repeat, this presence is essential, as long as it is subterranean; and because it is so, it is this experiential temporality that we want to talk about in this study, analysing its perception by humans as past, present and future.

The past would be the time that is moving away from us, from our consciousness, from our perception; it is everything that is no longer tangible, simply because it is gone. We call the present the "now", the time in which our experiences happen, at the moment they occur. And the future, in turn, corresponds to the set of events that will materialise as time passes. In other words, the future is like the place where all the facts that we will witness when a certain period of time elapses, no matter how short or long (OLIVEIRA, 2015).

Now, to speak of time as part of it implies having the "now" as a starting point, which is interesting to say the least if considered from the perspective of volume. What is the volume of the past? Most of our 'lived' life would fit within it, in other words, everything from now on would be placed within the past. The volume of the future would be just as equivalent, because from now on, everything is future.
From this perspective, how small and irrelevant the present becomes, no? Not even a full blink of our eyes could fit inside it.

Such reasoning makes it possible to realise that perhaps the linear or chronological division of time is not enough to explain it in all its complexity, much less to demonstrate it in people's lives. Humans are "beings in time", because we propose thinking of them from the perspective that it is in time that life takes place. As such, it is in the concreteness of lived reality that it gains meaning.

There's a Chinese proverb that says: "The past is history, the future is a mystery, and today is a gift. That's why it's called the present!" Now, can anyone say that life isn't an eternal amalgamation of stories and mysteries? - And many other things that can't even be counted.

In this context, authors deal with the 'time of the lived', attributing a dimension that distances itself from the sequenced form of distinct moments by which chronological time is marked; rather, it spreads through reverberations of experiences in which past-present-future move in spiral movements (DOLINA; BELLATO; ARAÚJO, 2014).

In this way, time can be thought of as a confluence in which the past and future "overlap the present", shaping it. The present, in turn, is an inexhaustible source of the lived, through which life gushes incessantly, letting the past pass through itself, while at the same time reflecting/reflecting, in "possibilities", the becoming, what we call the future.

In the present, we experience the future as an imagined expectation, in the sense of "looking forward" to a time that has not yet happened, but which is projected as something to be realised. In this way, the future is experienced through imagination, through the prospect of a created future that we try to live in the future, unlike what happens with the past, which is experienced through memory with re-significations in the present.

In this way, the present potentially carries with it the situations of the future world, it contains microscopic embryos that will develop and which are still invisible to our eyes (MORIN, 2010), but which already exist and cohabit "with" and "in" the present.

This embryonic cohabitation of the future in the present makes up the most intimate perspectives of human life and, we would venture to say, of each being's "happiness project". As it is in a shared life that the human being continues to project, and not alone, this is an interesting key to launching understandings, in this study, about the temporality of living in the family, a place where happiness projects cohabit.

In this reflection on time in the family experience, perhaps we can also envisage a notion of "legacy" as "what is left 'in' and 'for' the lives of those who remain". In this sense, the family is the maintainer of the legacy of moments of shared experience, with the "memory" of a family member being a bridge that makes possible their presence, which is absent in the physical world, but still has a place in the family body. In the introduction to his book "The Book of Hugs" (GALEANO, 2002), the author tells us that "to remember", from the Latin re-cordis, is to pass through the heart again. Thus, we can corroborate that there is an "absent presence" that remains in the family and is felt throughout life, affecting its dynamics and organisation (DOLINA; BELLATO; ARAÚJO, 2013).

Thus, we believe that the family provides care in such an integrative way that it is capable of encompassing "before birth", "during life" and "after life", transcending all the events that human beings experience. This is possible because of the affective relationship woven over time that, during life, shapes memories of shared moments, feelings and help. Thus, through the time lived and shared as a family, the loved one who is gone is never completely gone.

This lived and shared time is that which we feel, which is signified in the concrete of reality and which is before us from the moment we open our eyes until the moment we close them. It is variable, unstable and uncertain, conforming to the ways in which each person perceives and gives meaning to the present, combining it with their past and future anticipations (DOLINA; BELLATO; ARAÚJO, 2014).

Therefore, time is an organising dimension of human life and, in the midst of living, the chronic situation of illness is also expressed in temporalities that relate to the biographical daily experience, since it is lived differently by each person and each family. Becoming ill is therefore not limited to the chronology of the disease's evolution, nor to its clinical expression in periods of aggravation and stability (BELLATO et al., 2011).

Souza and Lima (2007) emphasise that chronic illness becomes part of a person's life for a prolonged or even indefinite period of time. We would also add that becoming ill is experienced as an experiential temporality (BELLATO et al., 2011) and that this is barely perceptible by health professionals and services, since care is organised and offered in strict protocol and institutional times, chronologically demarcated.

Getting sick is always a sensitive experience and, as such, the sense of duration can make a few minutes seem like a long time due to the subjective perception of its fullness and relevance (BACHELARD, 1994; BELLATO, 2001). In this way, the notion of duration is related to affective time, that which is experienced, felt and used by people. From this perspective, months, days and hours become much more like markers of experiences, all the more intense the more sensitive they are (DOLINA; BELLATO; ARAÚJO, 2014) than temporal units that account for chronological time.

Therefore, in this study, we are interested in exploring this contrast of times, despite the fact that the experience of falling ill in question has the characteristic of a precious present that stretches into uncertain tomorrows.

CHAPTER 5

COMPREHENSIVE APPROACH TO FAMILY EXPERIENCE AND RESEARCH PATHS

> The intimate understanding of objects is realised in the relationship with everyday life. It is poets and artists (even before theoreticians) who have this intuition (MAFFESOLI, 2008, p. 5).

This study is part of the comprehensive approach, which we see here as a creative way of doing research, which requires an open stance on the part of the researcher and the ability to give up one's own certainties in favour of the influences of reality (MINAYO, 2010). This reality is uncertain and inexhaustible in its complexity, given that

> [...] the world that people inhabit is made up of shapes, sounds, smells, textures, architectures, objects, movements, relationships - everything that can be apprehended by us, impressing our senses and intuitions. This world is therefore full of (un)sayables and (in)visibles; and it is a field of possibilities for the observer/researcher, requiring sensitive means of apprehension in research (BELLATO; ARAÚJO, 2015, p.1397).

Thus, understanding an event from the other person's perspective requires the researcher to adopt an understanding, sensitive and judgement-free stance. To this end, we consider it fundamentally important for the researcher to build a relationship with the study participant, mediated by the ethical values that both bring with them, with the researcher having to adopt an attitude of respect for people's ways of life and the meanings attributed to what they experience. Taking this stance implies admitting that research is intertwined with our own lives, so that in research we allow ourselves to be guided by what has acquired meaning and significance for us (CORAZZA, 2007).

In this sense, we worked with comprehensive research aimed at health and nursing, addressing the family experience of illness and care, realising that these experiences are lived in a unique and very personal way and can be known by us, even if only partially, through the narratives of people and their families.

These unfold in the logic of those who narrate, and it is up to us as researchers to try to understand them in their essence and context, taking as our presupposition that what is narrated conforms to the (re)interpretation and (re)meaning of what happened.

Therefore, in this study, we have deliberately taken on the task of trying to understand from the perspective of the other. To achieve this, we rely on authors who emphasise *the* sensitivity of the gaze in order to achieve 'eyes to see'. In this respect, we can learn from the advice of Rubem Alves (1999), who used to say that grandparents' eyes are wise because their characteristic is the ability to "taste" - in the sense of getting a flavour of something - and that this expands over the years.

Learning to "get to know" things requires sensitivity, time and a lot of willingness. With each effort to understand, the researcher's sensitivity to people's life situations also expands. The person who understands is, above all, the person who is sensitive to the events that permeate people's lives, as well as their own.

In an effort to bring out subsidies for a broader understanding of family care, within the framework of the matrix research group in which this study is included, all the stages of the scientific study are worked on in a shared manner, from the definition of the different work plans linked to it, the use of strategies and instruments in the field and the efforts to analyse the empirical material. This approach is taken collectively, so as to encompass the journeys, successes and mishaps in each study's own labour; and because it is considered that the exchange of experiences and reflections enhances research work and learning.

Furthermore, this way of proceeding enables the research group to exercise different skills and sensitivities during the research process, broadening the possibilities of understanding the family experience and, consequently, producing new knowledge with a view to changing professional practices.

Consistent with this understanding, the research group is organised into various work cells, each covering the history of a family and making up a Master's study, as well as two or three scientific initiation (CI) projects. In this case, the approach to Ricardo's family was therefore carried out by a work cell made up of myself, Juliana, master's student Ítala Paris de Souza and two CI students, Ariane Cristine de Carvalho and Camila de Oliveira Ribeiro, in a joint effort that brings together students at different stages of their training.

4.3 Methodological design of the study

This is a qualitative research study, as it requires the researcher to take an understanding stance towards the participants, allowing them to grasp the different meanings attributed by people to the processes they are experiencing (MINAYO, 2010).

It should be noted that qualitative research is characterised by empiricism and the progressive systematisation of knowledge until the internal logic of the group or process studied is understood, thus allowing for the construction of new approaches and the revision and creation of notions during the research process (MINAYO, 2010).

Considering that people experience the events in their lives in their own, very personal way, we chose to delineate it as a 'situation study' whose principle is to delve into the universe of everyday family life in an attempt to get to know it in depth (DOLINA; BELLATO; ARAÚJO, 2013), drawing some broader inferences from this micro-reality (MINAYO, 2010).

At the GPESC, the first approach to the "situation study" was Musquim's Master's Dissertation (2013), which highlighted care situations in the family context as important for understanding the experience of illness as a social process. The author based this on the notion of "situational analysis" proposed by Vai Vensen (2010), which presupposes more intense research in a smaller study unit, requiring greater emphasis in the field and in the presentation of data, as well as greater knowledge by the researcher of the subjects' personal histories and relationship networks.

The notion of a situation study, which we coined, has 'relationship' as its substantive element, in the sense that it aims to get to know the ways in which people and their families relate to each other, to other people, places, times, events and things, with our focus being the family experience of care in living and becoming ill. In this way, the situation study guides us to weave a close relationship with the family that makes it possible to perceive the personalities and singularities of their experience, apprehending sickness and care in the situation.

This experience, being unique, also transcends and touches the other person who, through the humanity emanating from the special situation, recognises themselves and empathises - not in the sense of putting themselves in their place, but in the desire to get to know them and become sensitive to the human experience of falling ill (BELLATO; ARAÚJO, 2015).

4.4 Meeting Ricardo's family

This study followed the inclusion criteria of the matrix research to which it is linked, which are: a) families living in the state of Mato Grosso, with the possibility of different family members taking part, including children, adolescents, adults and the elderly; b) being chronically ill; c) using public health services to some extent.

Based on these criteria, we called on a network made up of teachers and students from the Federal University of Mato Grosso, involved in different care situations, who could inform us about families who might meet these criteria.

A Master's student in Nursing presented us with the peculiar situation of a family that met the criteria for matrix research and also had some particularities of interest to the research group:

> *I learnt - through a first-year master's student - that there was a family experiencing a very rare illness and I was interested in finding out the story. It was about an 11-month-old baby, Ricardo, who was born with a syndrome called Schinzel-Giedion. This condition has imposed a number of changes on the life of the family, which is organising itself entirely to look after the child. I also learned that Ricardo's parents - Bruno and Jéssica - had gone* to court to get authorisation to use Cannabidiol, a medicine developed from cannabis leaves that reduces seizures and, as *a result, improves the baby's quality of life* (Observation notes - 11.06.2015).

Faced with the possibility of studying the family's experience of a rare illness, the parents' youth and the fact that Ricardo was the couple's first child, I was interested in getting to know the family, who were therefore intentionally chosen as participants in this study. We therefore recognise and value intentionality, since the researcher's personal nature is also involved when we approach human experiences that are so close to our existential reality with a sensitive and understanding attitude (PETEAN, 2013).

4.5 Research collection strategies and meetings with Ricardo's family

Different methodological strategies were used to understand the family experience, such as in-depth interviews and observation (ARAÚJO et al., 2013), in order to compose the life history of Ricardo's family.

Life History has enabled us to understand the way in which people tell their stories, in an endeavour to remember, in which the personal meanings they give to what they have experienced emerge, with varying intensities of their own, attributing importance to certain events in their lives (BELLATO et al., 2008; ARAÚJO et al., 2013).

The choice of the In-Depth Interview, understood as a dialogue with intentionality (MINAYO, 2010), was due to the fact that this strategy allows the person to speak freely about their experience, with the researcher's enquiries being guided in such a way as to gradually deepen certain narrative threads that emerge from the story, which presupposes several encounters in order to configure such depth in the interview (ARAÚJO et al., 2013).

Observation enabled us to grasp the unique contexts of life and care. In addition, this strategy allowed us to grasp the modes of expression that go beyond speech, marking ways of saying - orality; and the diversity of language - bodily, gestural, affective; along with the variable contexts in which dialogue takes place (ARAÚJO et al., 2013).

All the observation records, as well as the transcription of the narratives, made up the Research Diary, which is conceived by us as an important technology for recording and remembering events, taking shape as the research is carried out and allowing all the richness of the research process to be made visible (ARAÚJO et al, 2013). The use of the diary provides the researcher with a privileged space that allows them to give space to their voice and the way they relate to the field, being able to talk about their experience, observations and reflections on the moment of each meeting (ALVES, 2015).

When collecting the empirical material for this study, in an effort to preserve an atmosphere conducive to dialogue, we organised ourselves with the premise of not exceeding the comfortable number of people present at the meetings with the family; so we tried to take turns throughout the interview meetings, ensuring my participation in all of them, weaving the first and foremost bond with Ricardo's family. This took place according to a timetable with all the dates of the meetings and a rotation scheme between the CI students, so that two master's students and one CI student took part in each meeting with the family.

The interviews were recorded using the voice recorder app on the researchers' mobile phones, and we used three different devices positioned in strategic locations to capture the voices better.

The fieldwork lasted from June 2015 to January 2016. In the first month, we held weekly meetings with the family, trying to bring the research team closer to their care experience.

The first contact, mediated by a Master's student who already knew the family, was by telephone:

> Given this information about the family's living situation, I was very interested in getting to know them and I phoned Bruno, explained my study to him and asked if he and his wife would like to take part. He very kindly agreed and said he would explain it to his wife before giving me a final position. I called the next day and they agreed to take part in the study (Observation notes - 11.06.2015).

The first meeting was planned so that a schedule of subsequent meetings could be defined, and we made ourselves available to the family so that they could determine the best times and choose the place they preferred to hold them.

So, given the family's availability, we decided to meet every Thursday between 4.30pm and 5pm at the house where they live. Should any unforeseen circumstances arise, either on the part of the family or the research team, we would contact them and reschedule the date.

The first meeting at the family home took place on 11 June 2015 and, in order to describe it in more detail, here are excerpts from the observation records written at the time:

> The first meeting and the family's kind welcome
> We went in and soon I saw Jessica, who was in the corridor with her back to us, cradling Ricardo in her arms. I said: Jéssica? She turned to me and *we greeted each other. She's a very young girl - 24 years old - with dark skin and dark hair. She has a very cheerful countenance and was very welcoming to us. Ricardo is a small baby for his age, but it's not very noticeable that he suffers from a syndrome as aggressive as Schinzel-Giedion.* [...] *When we first arrived, he was crying a lot and seemed irritable, but as time went by and he was cuddled by his mum, he became calmer and even slept on her lap for a while.* [...] *After chatting a lot, the couple invited us to visit the other rooms in the house. I was surprised and delighted by their kindness. First we went to the bedroom where the couple's bed and Ricardo's cot are. The room was decorated in blue and white and behind the cot there were some knick-knacks made by Bruno's mum. I also remember some family photos on the wall.* [...] *The couple really opened their doors to welcome us in, sharing their history and way of life with us. They made a point of introducing us to every corner of where they live and the fact that this attitude happened at the first meeting and so spontaneously was very encouraging for me.* [...] *We were so well received that my initial impressions were the best, I felt a very harmonious relationship between Bruno and Jéssica, it seems that they form a couple who know how to "speak the same language". I found it interesting because, despite being so young, they seem to be mature enough to deal with their son's illness* (Observation notes - 11/06/2015).

So, from this first meeting onwards, subsequent weekly meetings were held, totalling eight so far, four of them at the family home and one at Ricardo's first birthday party, to which we were kindly invited by the family. This was an important occasion for us to correspond with the family who, keen for us to take part in this significant moment in their lives, opened up this privileged space for relationships, which we endeavoured to enter in an ethical and respectful manner.

> Ricardo's first birthday: Arraiá.
> The party, which was a charity event to raise funds for Ricardo's treatment, took place on a Saturday and was very well organised, there were more than two hundred people and the venue was very large.
> Right at the entrance, I spotted a wooden sign that read: Ricardo's Arraiá. At the door, a young man sat on a low chair with a table in front of him, he was wearing a big straw hat and was collecting the tickets. [...] The house where the party took place is very close to the federal university and has an extensive backyard with a large swimming pool. I don't know if anyone lives there or if it's just used for events. The whole place was decorated with colourful banners and there were some blue balloons in the pool. [...] When I arrived, Bruno and his mother-in-law were at the till. I chatted to them briefly as a small queue was forming behind me. Then I went over to Jéssica, who was sitting at a table with other people and was holding Ricardo on her lap. I greeted her, gave her the little souvenir I'd bought to celebrate Ricardo's birthday and introduced her to my mum. [...] Ricardo seemed very calm on his mum's lap, I put my hand on his head and wished him a happy birthday. [...] I noticed that there was a plastic cup on the table containing Ricardo's diet and Jéssica was using a syringe to feed him through the tube. [...] The party was a lot of fun, there were bands playing lively music and everyone was chatting a lot. [...] Next to the cashier were *cards with the prices - handwritten - of each product that could be bought at the party. They organised a token system, whereby the guest bought the token at the cash desk and could go to the stalls to collect sweets, food and drinks.* [...] *When we said goodbye, Bruno thanked us for coming and asked if everything was all right for Thursday, and I said yes. I was very happy with this question, because it seemed to me that they had some expectations of our meetings.* [...] *Jessica was extremely kind to us, thanked us for coming and also asked, in a very animated way, if we would be at her house on Thursday.* [...] *I was very happy to have the opportunity to be present at this moment in Ricardo and his parents' lives. I intend to talk a bit more about the organisation of the party at the next meeting, because from what I noticed, many people had mobilised their efforts to make it*

happen (Observation notes - 20.06.2015).

Since the beginning of the fieldwork, we have also communicated via *WhatsApp* messages, which has contributed to a certain extent to a relationship of prompt response and closeness between the author of this study and the family. With the family's authorisation, some of these messages were included in the Research Diary and therefore made up the *corpus* of analysis for this study, as well as the information collected from the online page maintained by the couple and some of the hospital documents provided by them.

4.6 The comprehensive path in research

We believe that the comprehensive research process involves transcribing the narratives, describing and interpreting the empirical material. These efforts were made from the first meeting with the family onwards, and were even necessary for the gradual deepening of the interview.

The process of transcribing the narratives is a moment of immersion in the family's life story, and is essential for understanding the experiences of illness and care. From this perspective, we refrained from using software specialised in transcribing and analysing data because we believe that human sensitivity is an essential element in this process.

Thus, at each meeting, the interview was transcribed meticulously and by hand by the work unit, and after it was finalised, the author of this study took care to listen to the audios again, trying to verify what had been transcribed and to add words that had not been noticed a priori. This transcription also included memories of the meeting, interspersing the speeches with descriptions that could give them a sense of context, such as gestures, silences, pauses, voice intonations and the events around us.

This artisanal labour involves the researcher adopting a 'seeing ear', who, in the coming and going of the recorded audios, in the pauses and repetitions, transfers to blank paper what he has 'seen' through his ears, as well as the feelings aroused by the speeches themselves and by the recollection of the meeting, trying to highlight aspects peculiar to the orality of each speech, even taking care with the ways of saying it, sometimes highlighting gestures, sometimes highlighting silences, in an attempt to preserve as much as possible the essence and intention of what was said (verbal information) .[6]

The Research Diary, containing all the field collection material and records of the research work, consists of 220 pages typed in a Microsoft Word Document (docx) file, in Times New Roman font, size 12 and single-spaced between the lines.

We read all this material carefully and thoroughly, colouring the narratives so as to differentiate them according to their meanings, which were then grouped and regrouped into axes of meaning. In a practical way, after colouring in the excerpts from the narratives, they were cut out and glued onto sheets of cardboard, thus constructing the first "analysis mats" of the study. Knowing that narratives follow the storyteller's own logic, the construction of the mats enabled a kind of ordering of the elements narrated, bringing together, in the space of the analytical drawing that was being formed, the narrative passages that interweave meanings.

[6] Ariane Cristine de Carvalho Brito, Cuiabá - MT, 2015.

In this way, the axes of meaning were gradually delineated through the intensive effort of approaching and distancing oneself from the empirical material. In this way, we corroborate the idea that the design of the research 'unfolds' gradually by giving certain reliefs to the complex fabric of human experience and this implies the sensitivity of the researcher in recognising the other and, also from this other, in being willing to make themselves known by revealing the meanings of the events that permeate their lives (BELLATO; ARAÚJO, 2015).

In addition, some clearer outlines of our understanding of the family experience are presented through descriptive-analysing images, in the form of drawings and diagrams. To this end, we refer to the construction of analysing diagrams in research that encompass such elements in order to systematise, synthesise and give visibility to the family experience of care and illness (MUSQUIM, 2013; COSTA et al., 2009; ARAÚJO et al., 2013).

The first drawing drawn up was "The family's search for professional care" which, because it was more descriptive, enabled us to delve into the narratives. It also gave rise to initial interpretations about the family's journey since Ricardo's birth, and was germinal to our enquiries about the time of this experience.

The second was the drawing of the "Family Genogram", which shows the nuclear conformation of Ricardo's family, as well as the relationships with other family members.

The third drawing was the "Spiral of Time", which emphasises the confluence of past, present and future, and in which the time lived by Ricardo's family is (re)signified. This drawing, which is more interpretative in nature, was reflected on in the research group's work meetings, so that the collective could emerge and converge in order to understand the different and varied times of life and care.

As a result of the comprehensive effort made in this study, we have chosen two axes of meaning that highlight significant dimensions of what this family experiences, and which are also expressive to them.

Thus, the axes of meaning of Ricardo's family's experience that emerged in this study are: a) caring in the situation of a rare illness: the family's experience and the ability of the health services to resolve it and b) re-significances and perspectives of the experience of having a child with the rare Schinzel-Giedion Syndrome. Emphasising these elements was possible due to the artisanal way in which we work, requiring the researcher to be sensitive to what people tell us and to perceive what they attribute in terms of meaning to the events they experience.

4.7 Ethical care in research with people and their families

The Brazilian guidelines for ethics in research with human beings consist of a set of resolutions from the National Health Council, embodied in Resolution No. 466/2012 (BRASIL, 2012).

This resolution serves as a guideline, with no pretence of precepting/prescribing conduct between humans in this situation. We therefore emphasise our respect for and compliance with the ethical prerogatives laid down, and the matrix research to which this study is linked was approved by the Ethics Committee of the Julio Muller University Hospital, under opinion No. 951.101/CEP-HUJM/2015.

The ethical sense with which we conducted this work is based, above all, on considering its humanistic, inter-relational and empathetic character (MINAYO; GUERRIERO, 2014).

Thus, we based ourselves on a few assumptions, such as the relationship between the researcher and the study participant, mediated by the ethical values that both bring with them; respect for the ways of life and meanings attributed to what people experience; careful conduct of the research, embodied in ethical values embodied in small acts, such as attentive listening, availability to be together, respect, reciprocity, empathy, little discussed in the research situation, but fundamental in the weaving of the researcher-participant relationship.

We would also like to point out that the family's participation was formalised by signing the Free and Informed Consent Form (FICF), at which point we assured them that their information would be confidential, guaranteeing secrecy throughout the research, including the dissemination of the results. At the time, the family gave us the freedom to use their real names:

> If you want to keep our normal name you can, you can. [...] Because ours is all public, our information. It's good that you ask us because there's a lot of wrong information. Then you sign again, right? (Jéssica, mum)

In this way, and with Bruno and Jessica's consent, we have only used fictitious names for institutions and people mentioned by the couple, respecting the family's wishes and the precept of anonymity. We also included an addendum to the ICF (APPENDIX II), formalising this choice.

Thus, we believe that human conduct is permeated by values that precede and guide ethical guidelines, and that it is up to the researcher to validate them in the research situation itself, which supports but goes beyond what is formalised in Resolution 466/2012. It is the researcher's challenge to show that the research situation, full of meticulous and essential care, presupposes sensitivity in order to instil unique ethical conduct.

CHAPTER 6

PRESENTATION OF RESULTS

The results presented here constitute a preliminary version of the manuscripts in accordance with the requirements of a qualified scientific journal in the area of Health and Nursing.

6.1 Caring for rare patients: the family's experience and the ability of health services to provide solutions[7]

INTRODUCTION

The family, regardless of its configuration, is a supporting pillar for the birth, growth and development of their loved ones, characterised as a place of mutual support where care for life and for life takes place (BELLATO et al., 2016). This means that the family offers care that goes beyond family relationships and encompasses the multiple dimensions of living, which makes it the main carer for each of its loved ones over time and generations. Family care is therefore considered by us to be broad and essential to life and health (GUITIERREZ; MINAYO, 2010).

In this sense, the onset of illness has repercussions on the life of the sick person, as well as those who are directly involved, care for them and are afflicted by their suffering (ALMEIDA; ARAÚJO; BELLATO, 2014). As illness is an intrinsic part of the movement of life and living, it requires the family to mobilise their care potential in a more intense way, especially when it is chronic, which can last for a long time or a lifetime.

This illness is highlighted in people's lives as a chronic situation, a term that seeks to broaden the view of the multiple contingencies that weigh on people and their families when they experience illness, as well as their concrete possibilities for caring for and being cared for (BELLATO et al. 2015). Therefore, this notion seeks to encompass the dynamics of becoming ill, caring and being cared for as a singular and personalised experience in the time-space of the family.

This study deals with the chronic situation caused by congenital illness, since there are peculiarities inherent in "being born sick", implying an intense re-signification by the parents, in terms of life and caring for their child. This situation takes on greater expression when the illness is a very rare syndrome that limits the child's time to live, giving the family a prospect of an uncertain future. Just like the family participating in this study.

The consequences that the rarity of an illness brings to the family carry with them specificities that are added to the illness. Parents often have to make immediate decisions about their child's treatment or face a

---

[7] From this manuscript came the article "Caring in the event of a rare illness: the family's experience and their search for support from health services", published in Revista Saúde e Sociedade, volume 25, number 4, 2016.

situation of lethality or disability that forces them to reshape their expectations (GONZÁLEZ-LAMUNO; FUENTES, 2008).

In the field of professional assistance, which is so necessary in rare disease situations, the discussion is relatively recent and has been gaining momentum in Brazil, especially since the enactment of Ordinance No. 199 of 30 January 2014, which establishes the National Policy for Comprehensive Care for People with Rare Diseases. This policy defines, in its article 3° , that "a rare disease is one that affects up to 65 people in every 100,000 individuals, i.e. 1.3 people for every 2,000 individuals" (BRASIL, 2014, p.3). Its aim is to

> [...] reduce mortality, contribute to the reduction of morbidity and mortality and secondary manifestations and improve people's quality of life, through promotion, prevention, early detection, timely treatment, reduction of disability and palliative care (BRASIL, 2014, p. 3).

To this end, it assigns responsibilities to the various state bodies, ranging from guaranteeing health services and human resources to monitoring mechanisms, with a view to improving the quality of actions (BRASIL, 2014). The Brazilian panorama, however, is still far from what is recommended in this document, with the scientific community and, above all, professionals working in health services still having limited knowledge of rare diseases. These factors contribute to the health system, in both its public and private dimensions, offering inadequate coverage for the needs of families experiencing this situation (PORTUGAL; ALVES, 2015).

We know that there are many elements that weigh on the care of people with rare diseases and the scientific studies that support professional health practices are still very limited in relation to this issue, making medical diagnosis, treatment and maintenance of care over time difficult, among other things. It is also noteworthy that the profiles of studies on rare diseases are mostly from the perspective of the clinical approach and are based on case studies of the disease.

There are still few studies on how a rare illness affects the lives of the sick person and their family, which is reflected in the possibility of supporting family care, as we will see in this study. Thus, the lack of knowledge on the part of health services and professionals about what a rare illness is, as well as how it can be controlled, contributes to increased anguish and suffering for the parents, promoting a certain 'disengagement' on the part of the family in their care.

In this sense, we consider this study to be an important contribution, as it was developed from the privileged perspective of a family experiencing the illness of their only child with the extremely rare Schinzel-Giedion Syndrome (SSG). This syndrome was described for the first time in 1978 by two researchers, Albert Schinzel and Andreas Giedion, and is characterised by an autosomal dominant genetic disorder (HOISCHEN et al., 2010) that causes numerous compromises to the life and health of the newborn.

Because it is a congenital, permanent and rare illness, SGA imposes an unexpected situation on parents when it comes to caring for their new family member. In this way, they have to make an intense and constant effort to find support of different kinds and in different places to help them provide the best care for their child. The family also has to deal with the seriousness of the illness and the knowledge of its lethality, which can lead to a cascade of feelings about their child and the uncertain tomorrow that lies ahead.

Thus, we aimed to understand the family's experience of caring for a child with a rare syndrome and to understand how health services and health professionals are able to provide solutions in terms of child care and family support.

METHOD

This is a study with a comprehensive approach, understood as the researcher's attitude towards the other, life and ways of knowing, in line with the way of understanding human beings in their incompleteness and impermanence (BELLATO; ARAÚJO, 2015). In line with this approach, the study was carried out from the perspective of a "situation study", the principle of which is to delve into the universe of everyday family life in an attempt to get to know it in depth (DOLINA; BELLATO; ARAÚJO, 2014), enabling us to draw some broader inferences from this micro-reality (MINAYO, 2010).

More generally, this study refers to the inclusion criteria of the matrix research to which it is linked, which are: a) families living in the state of Mato Grosso, with the possibility of different family members taking part, including children, adolescents, adults and the elderly; b) experiencing chronic illness; c) using public health services to some extent throughout the illness.

The participating family is made up of Bruno and Jéssica, a young couple aged 23 and 24 respectively, parents of Ricardo, who was born in June 2014 and was one year old at the time the empirical material was collected. Ricardo is the couple's only child and was born with SSG, a very rare, congenital, neurodegenerative disease with a sombre and uncertain prognosis.

In order to locate this family, we used a network of informants made up of nursing teachers and students from a public higher education institution in the state of Mato Grosso, who were involved in different care situations. Thus, given the possibility of covering the family's experience of a rare illness, the young age of the parents and the fact that Ricardo was the couple's first child, we were particularly interested in getting to know the family, which was therefore intentionally chosen to take part in this study. Thus, in advance, we recognise and value intentionality as a constituent and guiding element 'of' and 'in' research with a comprehensive approach, since the encounter with the other connects different stories and the researcher's personality is also involved when we approach human experiences that are so close to our existential reality with a sensitive attitude (BELLATO et al., 2016).

We corroborate that the research design 'unfolds' gradually by giving certain reliefs to the complex fabric of human experience; and this implies the researcher's sensitivity in recognising the other, and also the other's willingness to make themselves known, revealing the meanings of the events that permeate their life (BELLATO; ARAÚJO, 2015). So, in order to get to know this 'other' and understand the family's experience of care, we used different methodological strategies which, together, harmonise with our object of study.

The in-depth interview is understood as a dialogue with intentionality (MINAYO, 2010). It allows the person to talk freely about their experience, with the researcher's enquiries guided so as to gradually deepen certain narrative threads that emerge from the story (ARAÚJO et al., 2013). Together, we used observation, which enabled us to grasp the peculiar ways and contexts of life and care, as well as expression, which go beyond speech, and which encompasses and is interwoven with the variable contexts in which dialogue takes place (ARAÚJO et al., 2013).

Both strategies made up the Life Story of Ricardo's family, conceived by us as a privileged way of grasping the experiences of individuals and families, as it involves someone who 'tells' themselves to others and to themselves, and someone who listens to their experience and colours it, giving it relevance based on elements from their own experience (BELLATO; ARAÚJO, 2015).

All the observation records and full transcriptions of the narratives made up the Research Diary (ARAÚJO et al, 2013), consisting of 220 pages typed in a Microsoft Word Document (docx) file, in Times New Roman font, size 12 and single spacing between the lines. This information was collected between June 2015 and January 2016, totalling seven meetings. Of these, Bruno was present at four and Jéssica at all of them; during the first two months, we held weekly meetings with the family in an attempt to bring the research team closer to their care experience.

Understanding the empirical material involved delving into the family's narratives by carefully reading the entire research corpus, colouring the excerpts in order to differentiate them according to their meanings. In an effort to interpret this life experience, we tried to emphasise the elements most highlighted by the family, telling and retelling moments that they considered important in their experience of caring for their son. In this way, we emphasise that the family has referenced our "translation" of their experience in what they themselves have brought to our attention, which has proved to be validating for our efforts at understanding.

Through intense reflection on the empirical corpus, various axes of meaning emerged, including 'Search for specialised professional care and measures to relieve the symptoms of the syndrome'. Based on this, we sketched out some analysing drawings that reflected these searches for care, to which we related the time of Ricardo's life - in which we inquired about the time spent living and the specific interventions of the services. We then devised a first draft of the 'Lifeline of a child with a rare illness and the responses of the health services', which was presented to the family and complemented by them, with its various versions being gradually improved within the research group. According to Araújo and Lacerda (2008), drawings materialise mental images, constituting an interpretable sign as a representation of reality, showing that there is an intrinsic relationship between imagination and linguistic development.

We would like to emphasise that the timeline of Ricardo's first year of life was drawn up based on the family's narratives and consultation of documents provided by the hospital to the family, in order to cover the interventions of the health system and the times in which they occurred in the life of Ricardo and his family. In this way, the construction of this analytical design helped us to understand the elements that make up the axis of meaning in question. It also made it possible to present an image-synthesis of the time elapsed in Ricardo's life and, within it, the interventions of health services and professionals and, especially, the meanings attributed by the family to the situations that were unfolding with the arrival of their baby. This study respects and complies with the ethical prerogatives set out in Resolution 466/2012 (BRASIL, 2012), and the matrix research to which it is linked was approved by the Ethics Committee of the Julio Muller University Hospital, under No. 951.101/CEP-HUJM/2015. We would also like to emphasise that the family has given us the freedom to use the real names of the participants in this study. Therefore, with Bruno and Jessica's consent, we have only used fictitious names for institutions and people mentioned by the couple, respecting the family's wishes to be named, as well as the precept of anonymity for those mentioned.

RESULTS

The narratives of Ricardo's parents have shown us an intense pilgrimage through the various health services, calling on different professionals in an attempt to get some help in providing the best care for their son. Aware of the short life expectancy imposed by HGS, Jéssica and Bruno are extremely active, travelling beyond the geographical limits of the state where they live.

With the intention of giving visibility to this movement in search of resolutive professional care in a relatively short space of time, we present the 'Lifeline of a child with a rare illness and the responses of the health services'. This line is broken down month by month in order to provide a spatial grasp of Ricardo's life - just over a year - and to date the markers of important events in his follow-up by the various health professionals. To do this, we use capital letters of the alphabet, from A to L. We also present excerpts from the parents' narratives relating them to these markers, in order to explain the meanings attributed by the family to these events.

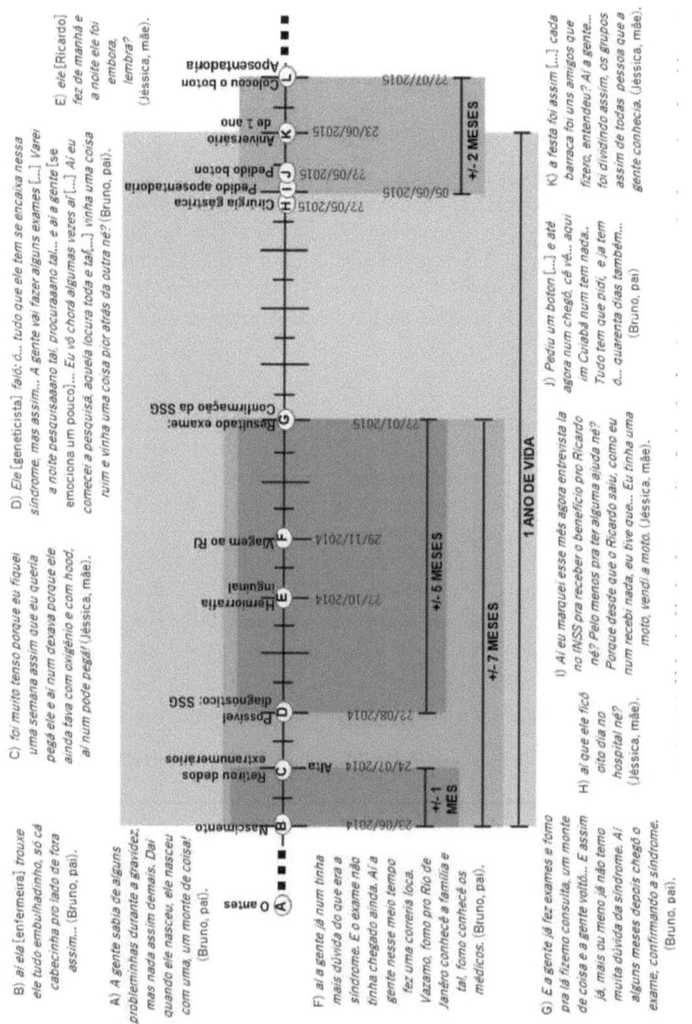

Figure 2: Lifeline of a child suffering from a rare illness and the responses of health services.

Even before Ricardo's birth, the couple received specific information about the possibility of their baby being born with some alterations (Figure 1, marker A). The first piece of news was the existence of a peculiarity in the umbilical cord, called a single umbilical artery. With subsequent prenatal consultations and ultrasound procedures, the couple also discovered other changes, such as polydactyly and alterations in the formation of the baby's kidneys and heart. Faced with this situation, the doctor in charge of Jéssica's prenatal care suggested that Ricardo might have a syndrome, which until then had been unknown to them.

Ricardo's birth (Figure 1, marker B) was a moment of great celebration and happiness for his parents and family, but it was also characterised by the time when assumptions left the realm of possibility and took centre stage in the concreteness of life:

> And then the nurse came to call me outside, in the reception area, and she said: "Ah Ricardo has been born, the baby has been born" and I said: "What's going on? No, everything's fine, it's just that the baby was born like this, like this"... full of problems! And then she asked if I wanted to see it, I said: "Of course! I want to see it, right? Then she said: "but it has to be very quick because he has to go straight to the ICU". (Bruno, father)

> He [Bruno] was already aware of things, I had nothing, right? Then I don't even remember the day I was hospitalised, the first day... I just remember that in the late afternoon, I wanted to see him [Ricardo] because I didn't really remember him, when he was born... Then I couldn't because I couldn't even stand up, and even if I could, I had to have showered to get into the neonatal ICU. So I couldn't see him the first day he was born. Then on the second day... the day he was discharged, I had a bath and went to see him... But he was so tiny, this little baby [he tunes his voice to speak in a very affectionate way]... (Jéssica, mum)

Due to numerous health problems, Ricardo's first month of life was spent in the Neonatal Intensive Care Unit (Figure 1, markers B-C). This was a period of great distress for his parents, who were in and out of hospital on a daily basis:

> [Thirty-four days in the ICU. [...] And then every day we had to go to the ICU, we went in the morning, afternoon and evening, right? [...] Oh yeah... I saw him more often... (Bruno, father). And it was necessary to take turns visiting, adjusting daily life to this demand, as Jéssica shows: [...] but at first I went with him [Bruno]. I only saw him [Ricardo] once, Bruno worked nearby. Then Bruno saw him twice, in the morning and in the afternoon. Then, as I was still undergoing surgery, he would only pick me up at certain times." (Jéssica, mother)

The difficulties went beyond what the couple had expected in terms of closeness and caring for their son, requiring both of them to re-signify their perspectives on parenthood in the face of the first demands of his illness. The technological artefacts that sustain and support Ricardo's life also stood in the way of this physical closeness and parental care, a situation that was poorly supported by the healthcare team in terms of minimising his suffering, since only the psychologist was more sensitive to this suffering, expressed in the mother's crying:

> After a fortnight I started, like after a week I picked him up. [...] Then I

> picked him up after a week when the psychologist saw that I was crying my eyes out, wanting to hold him... Then she went and asked to be released. [...] Then, after a week, I started trying to breastfeed him, right?
>
> [Jéssica stops speaking and continues to rub her son's face, then resumes speaking in a low tone of voice] So, it was one day that I tried, then the next day when I was going to pick him up, like this, to stay all day, he went back to the hood, so it was... I didn't pick him up for a few more days [speaks in a saddened tone]... (Jéssica, mum)

During the first year of his life, Ricardo also underwent three surgeries (Figure 1, markers C, E, H), the first of which was to correct and remove extranumerary fingers from his hands, the second an inguinal herniorrhaphy and the third a gastric surgery with fundoplication:

> He's already had three operations [...] so, poor thing... he was born with six little fingers on both hands, so we took them off [laughs] [...] that one he had in the ICU [laughs]. And then, soon afterwards... He was born with his testicle up here, it hadn't finished descending, so he had an inguinal hernia. And the hernia kept going down, it was occasional, right? Then it started going down all the time and there was a ball here [shows lower abdomen], everything swelled up... Then we had the operation too. He had three stitches here [points to the area of the abdomen where the incision was made]. And then he had the gastro, now [...] and the gastro was a bit more delicate because it was with a fundoplication, if it was just the gastro it would have been done quickly... (Bruno, father)

The surgery to remove the supernumerary fingers meant more than just correcting a problem that could cause Ricardo some motor difficulties, as it was also an aesthetic concern on the part of the parents in relation to their son, in an effort to achieve a certain body normality. The decision for the herniorrhaphy and gastric surgery procedure was made because it would benefit Ricardo's growth and development, in the sense of providing him with relief and comfort for a better life. Jéssica and Bruno continue, with each decision to be made, to weigh up the proportional gains for Ricardo and, as such, sometimes decide to forego procedures that could cause him suffering, as expressed in the following extract: He was born with hypospadias too... But he pees and urinates normally... so we've ruled out this surgery. We're not even going to do it anymore because it's delicate, right? So it's suffering for him, it's not a necessity... It's more aesthetic than necessary (Bruno, father).

After this first month in hospital, Ricardo was discharged from the maternity hospital (Figure 1, marker C) and the couple were able to take their son home; however, they carried a lot of uncertainty and anguish with them, as they didn't know exactly what their son's health conditions were. This was an intense period of "examination-consultation", which shows the agonising search for a diagnosis:

> Then... we came out of the ICU, a lot of doctors started... Wow, we went to 10 or 12 doctors... You know... I stopped my life, her life [Jéssica] and I was running around every day. Every day, check-ups, check-ups. And then his little problems started appearing... and then we started adapting. So, that's when we started seeing a geneticist [...] until then, we knew that he was not normal, that he had a few problems, we didn't know what, right? (Bruno, father)

The couple's intense search for professional attention was also focused on the symptoms Ricardo presented and how to care for him as he developed and the consequences of his illness progressed. However, they didn't see any similarities between Ricardo's situation and that of other sick children; nor did the doctors recognise any clinical cases that could serve as a reference. In the midst of trial, error and success, the geneticist who accompanied Ricardo suggested a possible diagnosis (Figure 1, marker D) to be confirmed by a specific test of partial sequencing of one of the segments of the mutated gene - exon 4 of SETBP1, and the result was obtained after ninety days:

> [...] we went there and made the enquiries and so on and a month later... he called us there, right? When we got there, he opened the book that he'd studied, researched a lot, written there... the book was all in English. He said: oh... everything he has fits into this syndrome, but... We're going to do some tests and stuff and... Then, like... at the weekend, on Friday, he started having these spasms... and we thought it was a break. It was all: "Oh, it's a break, it's a break...". Well, it would have been, wouldn't it? Then we got there and started to get a bit bigger, then we got there and went to tell him [the geneticist] about it. He said: Ah, the first thing that appears in the syndrome here is CONVULSION! [...] Then he went to research the place that tested for the syndrome, right? there were only three laboratories in São Paulo... and we went to research it... [...] Ninety days to send the results of the test... (Bruno, father).

Anticipating the diagnosis of SSG, Jéssica and Bruno mobilised themselves in search of information about the syndrome and everything they could find out about it. They found only two cases of the syndrome in Brazilian children through an internet search, and then contacted their families online and by telephone:

> Then we found, we discovered two little children here in Brazil who had... one in Rio de Janeiro and the other in Bahia. Then I tried to get in touch with the family and so on and I couldn't, it took a few days. Then Mininho's father, from Rio de Janeiro, created a website... that's where I found out everything, most things and so on. So I tried to get in touch

> with him, sent him a message on the site and so on, and a few days later they replied. [...] Theirs had... died aged two years and four days, in Rio... Two years and four days, right? And then we managed to get in touch too... We got in touch with his family in Bahia. Then... he'd died a month earlier too... [she speaks very emotionally, like she's trying not to cry. She remains silent for a while and then resumes] So, it was the two we knew, right? [Silence] That was an even bigger shock! (Bruno, father).

Jéssica and Bruno obtained support from two families, as well as a lot of information about the syndrome and its physical repercussions. They were also able to recognise their own experiences in situations very similar to those experienced by the families as a result of GHS. This recognition motivated the families to share knowledge and care, difficulties, afflictions and perspectives - which was very important for Ricardo's parents to see the 'best care' for their son.

Whilst it brought comfort to Jéssica and Bruno, the knowledge that the two children had already died provoked feelings of distress about how long their son would live. For the parents, the mismatch between their expectations and the reality that was unfolding in relation to Ricardo in his first year of life was due to the premature death of the children of the two families they contacted, including the vivid suffering at this moment of encounter.

This reality also contrasted with the normal markers of child growth and development, to which Ricardo did not conform. Faced with this, rather than being in a hurry, the family had an urgent need to look after Ricardo, anticipating his needs. This same urgency meant that he had to be cared for from a medical perspective, based on clinical practice and knowledge.

So, trying not to waste the valuable time of their son's life, Bruno and Jessica decided, at the invitation of the family in Rio de Janeiro (Figure 1, marker F), to meet in person and find out more about the situation they were beginning to realise they would be experiencing with their son:

> Then, like this, he grew up, the problems started to appear and so on... and then we no longer had any doubts about what the syndrome was. And the test hadn't arrived yet. So in the meantime, we went on a mad rush. We left, we went to Rio de Janeiro to meet the family and so on, to meet the doctors. That's where we met his doctor today, his neurologist is from there... [...] And we had our tests and went there for a consultation, a lot of things and we came back... And so, more or less, I no longer had much doubt about the syndrome. Then a few months later the test came back, confirming the syndrome... (Bruno, father)

From the point of view of the health professionals, the time taken for the diagnostic confirmation of the existence of the very rare syndrome can be considered relatively short: from Ricardo's birth to the diagnostic suspicion listed by the geneticist, two months passed (Figure 1, marker B to D); from then until the confirmation of the HGS, five months passed (Figure 1, marker D to G); and then, seven months after the child's birth, the diagnosis was confirmed (Figure 1, marker B to G).

However, in the seven months they lived and shared with Ricardo, aware of the immeasurable value of 'time' in his life, the family anticipated the result of the confirmatory SSG test and tried, through their own personalised means, to learn about the situation of his illness and to put together the conditions to take better care of him. Among these conditions, we highlight Ricardo's requests for retirement and for the boton to be placed in his gastrostomy (Figure 1, markers I, J), which took around two months to be answered positively (Figure 1, marker L).

It's also worth mentioning Ricardo's one-year birthday party (Figure 1, marker K) on 23 July 2015, which was celebrated by his family, friends and some of the professionals who work with him, making it an occasion to celebrate life and victory over the difficulties faced by the family. The party was also important for raising funds for Ricardo's treatment, as the health insurance contracted by his parents doesn't fully cover all the treatment required due to his illness.

CHAPTER 7

DISCUSSION

Families take care of their loved ones in a broad way, encompassing the multiple dimensions of living (BELLATO et al., 2016). This care is permanent and lasts throughout time and life cycles, from birth, through maturity and old age, until death; in this way, the family provides answers to the needs of their loved ones of all kinds. However, attention must be paid to the care potential available to them, given that this is limited and/or can be exhausted, as in situations that last over time, including the rare chronic illness experienced by the family in this study.

The family also draws on its care networks and searches to provide the best for their sick loved one. These searches are not restricted to a specific formalised institutional space (BELLATO et al., 2009), but go beyond it in order to find a solution to their needs.

In this sense, Ricardo's family seeks to offer the 'best care' and, in order to provide it, they mobilise themselves in a way that goes beyond institutional protocols and predictive behaviours, involving a complex process of interpretations and intuitions about their son's health situation. This process involves realising and sensing, or 'anticipating' - in the sense of anticipating - what will be beneficial for Ricardo.

The 'best care' involves weighing up what is the most convenient, sensible, prudent and right thing to do with Ricardo, and the parents' decision making takes into account a complex web of elements - especially the time of his life - which are judged in the situation and materialised in line with each need he presents, as well as all of them, taken as references. These considerations are considered and discussed by the parents in order to integrate possibilities for living well and reducing the suffering resulting from Ricardo's illness.

In this way, we see care that unfolds 'from, in and for' the child's life, seeking to leave them well within the possibilities that present themselves in the present - here and now -, not allowing finitude, although it may present itself as near, to be a deadly and limiting horizon (BELLATO, ARAÚJO; 2015).

This family's experience teaches us that care takes place 'in life' because it is provided in the midst of daily life itself and involves a keen eye that parents develop over time, capable of perceiving the 'minuteness' of their child's needs. Care is also 'for life', as it aims to promote the best conditions for living well and happily, thus distancing itself from the idea of care restricted to getting sick. Caring 'for life', in turn, has even broader dimensions, projecting itself towards tomorrow, involving the dreams and expectations that parents have for their child's life and future.

Since it is in the life shared in everyday life that human beings continue to project themselves in their continuous becoming, it encourages us to reflect on the temporality of family life, a place where happiness projects are built and shared. We agree with the author (AYRES, 2011) on the notion of happiness as a lived and positively valued experience that is independent of what is conventionally considered to be complete well-being or perfect morphofunctional normality.

The family thus seeks to embrace Ricardo's unique normality, which differs from other children his age, dealing with his peculiarities and daily needs in shared life. Authors (SOUZA; LIMA, 2007) emphasise that illness, especially chronic illness, brings with it the creation of new normalities in people's lives, different from the previous one. These normalities help people to cope with the chronic situation of illness, as they increase their chances of living better and being happier.

However, Ricardo's own way of being and living is also a strong element of 'differentiation' and, in view of this, his parents try to accept with a certain tranquillity the gazes and impressions of other people who don't live with him, in an attempt to minimise discomfort in relation to 'being different', thus reducing suffering related to a situation where their child doesn't fit in with the standards imposed as 'normal', both by health professionals and by society in general. We would like to emphasise that although this differentiation is quite marked, structurally and functionally, by health professionals in terms of the parameters of normality, whether in terms of growth or development of children with rare syndromes, it does not seem to receive the same reception in order to produce and provide care in line with their needs, in other words, distinctive to their personalities, and does not always generate greater effectiveness in professional practices through the application of positive discrimination.

In a very important way, the temporality of these children's lives needs to be taken into account when providing health care, in other words, to the extent and in the time required by the needs they present, expanding, to a certain extent, the resolution capacity of health services. A study on the family experience of caring for an adolescent with adrenoleukodystrophy already warned of the importance of considering worsening health needs, given that it is a degenerative disease, so that the care offered is progressively renewed over time and professionals are able to support families in this care (NEPOMUCENO et al., 2012).

The family recognises Ricardo's own normality based on other children, sharing experiences with other families who have also experienced a similar illness, which has provided essential support and help to better deal with their son's situation. We would like to stress that recognising the singularities in their child's way of becoming ill is fundamental in shaping the provision of care, as this is how the family organises itself to offer what the child needs (PETEAN; ARAÚJO; BELLATO; 2016).

We therefore propose a reflection here: what considerations can be made about the resolutiveness of the practices offered by health services and professionals for this child who is experiencing a very rare and life-limiting illness?

It's possible to find some paths by observing the family's care methods. Jéssica and Bruno provide all the care required by Ricardo's young age; and, concomitantly and intertwined, those required by the SSG itself stand out. In this confluence of intense, continuous and permanent care to sustain life, we can see the parents' acute concern about the 'time that passes', given that this is a syndrome that shortens their son's life expectancy. The development of care that encompasses and integrates their son's needs is therefore being worked out in situations, i.e. with each need presented by Ricardo, the parents jointly consider the best course of action to remedy it.

Thus, the complex range of care offered by the family, whether aimed at responding to the needs of the child at a young age, or that generated by the illness, is painstakingly woven together in an integrative way, focussing on Ricardo's well-being and his development in whatever way possible. This integrative perspective is a far cry from that of health services and professionals who, in turn, offer strictly ad hoc responses, since they are directed at what is required at a given moment, with little anticipation of what will be needed or a broader perception of the set of needs that "being a child" and "being seriously ill" generate.

We can see, then, that quite different logics guide health professionals and families when it comes to offering care. While the latter seek a possible solution to the needs imbricated in the daily routine of living and caring, health services/professionals offer a certain capacity to resolve "health problems" cut out from the broader list of needs that illness imposes (BELLATO et al., 2009).

Thus, to the extent that the services and professionals offer responses that are still not very resolute to the needs demanded by Ricardo's illness, his parents' efforts to weave support networks that can guarantee them a degree of effective care, albeit in other ways, are greatly increased. In this respect, authors emphasise that when faced with partial responses from the health service, in which people don't get the solution they need for their problems, this situation becomes the "driving force" for undertaking other care-seeking paths (BELLATO et al., 2009).

We realise, then, that everyday life and the constant threat posed by the syndrome call for more urgent solutions than the services and professionals can - and are willing - to offer. The family, in turn, takes advantage of and maximises Ricardo's time in life, seeking out knowledge about SSG on their own in order to find possible solutions for caring for their son in full. In this way, the element of 'time' takes on special importance, since it is in time that Ricardo's life takes place, and it is also in time that the suffering of the uncertain tomorrows imposed by the very rare SSG dwells.

Time, therefore, has valuable meaning in the reality lived and shared as a family, and it is up to Jéssica and Bruno to create and recreate the 'best care' for their son on a daily basis in order to maximise his time of life. And for the parents, "maximising Ricardo's time to live" means both extending it as much as possible and offering quality life in that possible time. Time therefore takes on the meaning of temporality, because it is affective time that is afflictively lived in its inexorable flow, and must therefore be enjoyed intensely. This affliction, which has the character of "anguished tribulation", does not close in on itself as annihilating pain; quite the opposite, it forges perseverance, as it aims for the horizon of hope; this resides in the very being of the son, Ricardo, and also in Jessica and Bruno, in the parents they long to be.

From this perspective, authors (DOLINA; BELLATO; ARAÚJO, 2014) deal with 'temporality' by attributing a dimension that distances itself from the sequenced form of distinct moments by which chronological time is marked. Instead, it spreads through reverberations of experiences in which past-present-future flow in spiral movements.

Therefore, time is an organising dimension of human life and, in the midst of living, the chronic situation of illness - especially rare, congenital and degenerative illness - is also expressed in temporalities that concern the biographical daily experience, since it is lived differently by each person and each family. Becoming ill is therefore not limited to the chronology of the disease's evolution, nor to its clinical expression in periods of aggravation and stability (BELLATO et al., 2011). On the contrary, it occurs in the context of 'experiential temporality', which refers to lived and shared time, that which we feel/signify in the concrete of reality and which is before us from the moment we open our eyes until the moment we close them.

This experiential temporality (BELLATO et al., 2011) ends up being barely perceptible to health professionals and services, since organised care is offered in strict protocol and institutional times, chronologically demarcated. On the other hand, the time lived is variable, unstable and uncertain, taking shape in the ways in which each person perceives and gives meaning to the present, combining it with their past and future anticipations (DOLINA; BELLATO; ARAÚJO, 2014).

Therefore, in order to increase their capacity to provide solutions, health services and professionals also need to set in motion different notions of time and temporality in order to reconsider the protocol-based and rigidly formalised times that, as a rule, guide their actions and the organisation of care processes, in an effort to embrace the temporality of living with and caring for children

with other normalities. So let's think again: what are two months of waiting for a child like Ricardo?

Ricardo has multiple, differentiated needs, as well as being marked by his unique temporality, which in itself should mobilise agile, precise and effective responses; however, even the guarantee of his rights, which are already formally guaranteed, has followed the logic of the institutionalised flow of demands in the services that have to respond. If the pension is intended to offer some financial support for Ricardo's possible and limited lifetime, two months of waiting have gone by. It would be important for the bureaucratic procedures for this demand to take into account the time of life that is being shortened by the very severity imposed by the SSG on this child.

Furthermore, the time taken to confirm the diagnosis of a very rare syndrome, such as HGS, may be considered quick by health services/professionals. However, it is in stark contrast to the temporality experienced by the family as they live through each day that begins and ends, permeated by uncertainties about the next day, worrying about a time that is projected into uncertain tomorrows, which they have had to learn to deal with on their own.

We therefore understand that health services and professionals are faced with major challenges when offering professional care, since the practices produced in this area need to synergise with family care, reinforcing and expanding their potential (SILVA; BELLATO; ARAÚJO, 2013), and not exhaust them by increasing the effort to seek effective care at the right time for their needs.

CHAPTER 8

CONCLUSION

This study seeks to incite important reflections, based on the many lessons that the family provides us with about their very personal way of caring "for, about and in life", as well as the partial and fragmented responses that professional health practices offer them to the ever-expanding and renewed needs of their child. Developed in the form of a 'situation study' of a young couple experiencing the illness of their only child due to a rare and life-limiting syndrome, we do not lend ourselves to generalisations, but stress that people's lived experiences have the human dimension at their core and that this cuts across different family experiences.

The parents care with a keen and expanded sense of care that flows in different directions, spreading throughout Ricardo's life, encompassing and integrating his needs in order to respond to them in the best possible way. On the other hand, health professionals have a diffuse perception, which takes Ricardo within the scope of his "shelf life", as his father "dolefully" expressed to us, and generally produces a feeling of disappointment and hopelessness in the family, given that there is so much to be done in caring for their son affected by the extremely rare and lethal syndrome.

And in order to find hope again, the family endeavours to get closer to other families who are experiencing or have experienced a similar situation, learning and teaching them very personal ways of looking after their most precious possession - their child's life - in their own normal way and in the flow of time that is possible.

Faced with a syndrome whose characteristic is to compromise life expectancy in its early years, it is essential that families are supported by health services and professionals in order to offer resolutive responses in the shortest possible time. And if time is running out, it is all the more important to offer expanded, precise and effective professional practices that are based on living, and not just on the deadly commitment of the disease.

The resolution capacity of health services is of paramount importance and needs to be rethought, weighing up the protocol times in the field of health against the different temporalities of each person's life. In Ricardo's situation, the shortness and unpredictability of the time 'of and in' life prompt reflection on how services have managed to support families, taking into account the normalities they experience.

We need to reflect on this rapid chronological time that shortens life chances if it is not used efficiently and effectively to meet their unique needs. Therefore, services need to do more than offer answers to specific problems, they need to support families in their needs in order to support them in this care that is so minutely modelled by them.

In this sense, in 2013, Brazil experienced an encouraging opportunity to advance knowledge and support for families living with rare diseases, hosting the 1st Ibero-American Congress on Rare Diseases, which represented an opportunity for dialogue between patients, carers, representatives of civil associations, the Ministry of Health, the legislature, researchers and academics. In this way, it was possible to broaden horizons towards new perspectives for approaching rare diseases, in order to decentralise the traditional discussion on clinical and drug treatment.

Also, due to the necessary limitation of the focus of this study, other dimensions of the family's experience of caring for their child with a rare syndrome were not explored. However, they give rise to important reflections and also concern the restricted resolutiveness of health services, such as the multiple costs that the family incurs in order to provide the best care for their child and which remain, as a rule, in the order of the barely visible, be they material, social, emotional, psychological, among others, that come from caring.

REFERENCES

ALBANO, L. M. J. et al. Hydronephrosis in schinzel-giedion Syndrome: an important clue for the diagnosis. Rev. Hosp. Clin. Fac. Med. S. Paulo, v. 59, n. 2, p, 89-92, 2004.

ALMEIDA, K. B. B.; ARAÚJO, L. F. S.; BELLATO, R. Family care in the experience of a young person's chronic illness. Rev Min Enferm. v. 18, n. 3, p.724-32, 2014.

ARAÚJO, L. F. S. et al. Research diary and its potential in qualitative research. Revista Brasileira de Pesquisa em Saúde, v. 15, n. 3, jun./set. 2013.

ARAÚJO, C. C. M.; LACERDA, C. B. F. Examining children's drawing as a therapeutic resource for the language development of deaf children. Rev Soc Bras Fonoaudiol. v. 13, n 2, p. 186-92, 2008.

AYRES, J. R. C. M. Care, ways of being (human) and health practices. In: AYRES, J. R. C. M. (Org.). Care: work and interaction in health practices. 1ª ed. Rio de Janeiro: CEPESC: UERJ/IMS: ABRASCO, 2011. p. 75-105. 284p.

BRAZIL. National Health Council. Approves regulatory standards for research involving human beings. Resolution no. 466, 12 December 2012. Lex: Federal Official Gazette. 2012

Jun.:01-52.

BELLATO, R.; ARAÚJO, L. F. S. Towards a comprehensive approach to the family care experience. Cienc Cuid Saude, v. 14, n. 3, 2015.

BELLATO, R. et al. Family experience of care in chronic situations. Rev Esc Enferm USP, 2016. PRELO

BELLATO, R. et al. Therapeutic itineraries of families and networks for care in chronic conditions: some assumptions. In: PINHEIRO, R;

MARTINS, P. H. (Orgs.). Health evaluation from the user's perspective: a multicentre approach. 1ª ed. Rio de Janeiro: CEPESC/IMS-UERJ; Recife: Editora Universitária UFPE; São Paulo: ABRASCO, 2009. p.187- 194. 376 p.

BELLATO, R. et al. Mediation and mediators in the therapeutic itineraries of individuals and families in Mato Grosso. In: PINHEIRO, R.; MARTINS P. H. (Orgs.). Users, social networks, mediations and integrality in health. Rio de Janeiro: CEPESC/IMS-UERJ; Recife: UFPE, São Paulo: ABRASCO, 2011. p. 177-83

BRAZIL. Ministry of Health. Ordinance No. 199 of 30 January 2014. Approves the National Policy for Comprehensive Care for People with Rare Diseases. Federal Official Gazette. 2014.

CARVALHO, E. et al. Schinzel-Giedion syndrome in two Brazilian patients: Report of a novel mutation in SETBP1 and literature review of the clinical features. American Journal of Medical Genetics. v. 167, n. 5, p. 1039-46, 2015.

DOLINA, J. V.; BELLATO, R.; ARAÚJO, L. F. S. Distinct temporalities in the breast cancer disease process. Rev. esc. enferm. USP, v. 48, n.2, p. 73-80, 2014.

GERHARDT, T. E. et al. Sensitive criteria for measuring the repercussions of professional care on the lives of individuals, families and communities. In: PINHEIRO, R.; SILVA JUNIOR, A. G. (Org.). Por uma sociedade cuidadora. 1. ed. Rio de Janeiro: CEPESC/IMS-UERJ/ABRASCO, 2010. chapter XX, p. 293-306 10.

GONZÁLEZ, L. D.; FUENTES, M. G. Rare diseases in paediatrics. An. Sist. Sanit. Navar. v. 31, supl. 2, p. 21-29, 2008.

GONZÁLES, L. V. et al. Schinzel-Giedion syndrome: new mutation in SETBP1. An Pediatr (Barc), v. 82, n.1, p. 12-16, 2015.

GUTIERREZ, D. M. D.; MINAYO, M. C. S. Production of knowledge on health care within the family. Ciência e Saúde Coletiva, v. 15, sup. 1, p. 1497-508, 2010.

HOISCHEN, A. et al. De novo mutations of SETBP1 cause Schinzel- Giedion syndrome. Nature Genetics, v. 42, n. 6, p. 483-85, 2010.

MINAYO, M. C. S. O desafio do conhecimento: pesquisa qualitativa em saúde. 12 ed. São Paulo: Hucitec, 2010.

NEPOMUCENO, M. A. S. et al. Ways of weaving networks for care by families living with chronic adrenoleukodystrophy.
Cienc Cuid Saude, v. 11, n. 1, p. 156-65, 2012.

PETEAN, E.; ARAÚJO, L. F. S.; BELLATO, R. Space-time dimension and the acts-attitudes of care in the family experience, 2016. J. res.: fundam. care. PRELO.

PORTUGAL, S.; ALVES, J. P. Rare diseases and care: a look at social networks. In: IBEROAMERICAN CONGRESS ON RARE DISEASES, I, 2015, city. Proceedings. Coimbra: Centre for Social Studies - University of Coimbra, 2015. p. 34-40.

SILVA, A. H.; BELLATO, R.; ARAÚJO, L. F. S. Daily life of the family experiencing the chronic condition of sickle cell anaemia. Revista Eletrônica de Enfermagem, v. 15, n. 2, p. 437-36, 2013.

SOUZA, S. P. S.; LIMA, R. A. G. Chronic condition and normality: towards the movement that expands the power to act and be happy. Rev Latino-am Enfermagem, v. 15, n. 1, 2007.

6.2 Resignifications and perspectives of what was lived in the experience of having a child with the rare Schinzel-Giedion Syndrome

INTRODUCTION

This study deals with the family's experience of caring for and being disabled by a very rare syndrome called Schinzel-Giedion syndrome (SSG), an autosomal dominant genetic disorder (HOISCHEN et al., 2010) that is congenital and neurodegenerative, causing numerous impairments and limiting life expectancy to the first few years. In contrast to clinical studies dealing with rare diseases (GONZÁLES et al., 2015; CARVALHO et al. 2015), we sought to highlight the perspective of what is experienced by a family made up of a young couple, Jéssica and Bruno, and their baby Ricardo; and, in this experience, the meanings of an 'original normality' experienced in relation to the only child born with the syndrome.

This perspective of normality, referenced in the experience of Ricardo's parents, encourages us to reflect on the different being of the child born with SSG, as they see it, as full of potential that needs to be exercised, within the best conditions they can offer them, with a view to their fulfilment as a child in the time of their life.

This understanding aims to deconform the precarious notion that takes the limited 'life span' as the limit of one's own 'being and living', in which the child is considered to be unviable and/or disabled. As a rule, disability is usually understood in relation to its opposite - through the particle "of", with the 'efficient' being its identity referent, even though it cannot be, which conforms it as a 'being of lack'. So, we propose that there is an original normality of the child born with a rare syndrome, such as SSG, to be perceived in itself, because it refers to the possibilities of its being a child; of course, it is not very productive to contrast it with the defining standards of what is 'normal' for children of the same age, such as those of "child growth and development".

In approaching a notion of disability, we start with the Brazilian Law on the Inclusion of People with Disabilities (BRASIL, 2015, p. 20), whose definition raises the nature of the person's impediments in relation to time and the barriers to their participation in society:

> A person who has a long-term physical, mental, intellectual or sensory impairment which, in interaction with one or more barriers, may hinder their full and effective participation in society on an equal basis with others.

However, we tried to look at another way of perceiving disability and, in the family experience we discussed, we highlighted the intense confluence of 'getting sick' in living, since the baby, having been born with the syndrome, is the "normality" possible in his life, and it is 'with and for' this different being that the parents shape their ways of living and caring.

On the one hand, being conceived and born with impairments and limitations in their lives brings with it various new meanings for the parents in relation to their child; on the other hand, a syndrome that limits the child's own life span, permanently compromising it in the early years, greatly emphasises the persevering and hopeful movement of the parents in living Ricardo's original normality, welcoming him and caring for him.

Authors emphasise the impact of the medical and social meaning of being outside the norm and how this marks the lives of rare disease patients and their families, with this normativity being revealed in the body, implying furtive glances and avoided contacts (PORTUGAL; ALVES, 2015). On the other hand, Souza (2006) states that there are various "normalities" present in the different ways of going through life, showing them to be flexible, dynamic and changeable. And in relation to living with chronic illness, authors emphasise people's ability to deal with the challenges that arise, overcoming them in such a way as not to restrict their ways of going through life (SOUZA; LIMA, 2007). Thus, we aimed to understand the resignifications and perspectives of the experience of having a child with the rare Schinzel-Giedion Syndrome.

The scientific contribution of this study comes from the fact that it was developed from the perspective of the family experiencing the situation of rarity due to SSG, following a different logic to that which has discussed it, centred on the clinical and diagnostic spheres. Furthermore, by encompassing the perspective of a family that engenders care geared towards their child's specific needs, we hope to provide support so that health professionals can offer protective practices to families experiencing rare syndromes, in order to strengthen them in their care potential, supporting them in coping with situations arising from the original normality of their loved ones.

In this sense, we emphasise that health services have a lot to learn from family experiences of care, especially when it comes to rare disorders, since the family is the main provider of care for their loved ones, whether they are ill or not. As an encouraging prospect for progress in this discussion, we highlight the 1st Ibero-American Congress on Rare Diseases, which problematised the need to consider models of care in the health system in which the person is the centre of all attention and discussions about rare diseases and drug treatment is just one of the ways, among others, needed to guarantee quality of life.

METHODOLOGY

This is a comprehensive study developed from the perspective of the 'situation study', which guides us to look at the daily life of the family in an effort to get to know it in more depth (DOLINA; BELLATO; ARAÚJO, 2013) and, from this micro-reality, draw some broader inferences (MINAYO, 2010).

With this in mind, we sought to include the family taking part in this study, made up of Bruno and Jéssica, a young couple - 24 years old, parents of Ricardo, born in June 2014, one year old at the time the empirical material was collected. Ricardo is the couple's first and only child and was born with SSG.

We located this family through a network of informants made up of nursing teachers and students from a public higher education institution in Mato Grosso, who were involved in different care situations. The family was chosen intentionally because of the possibility of getting to know the family's experience of a rare illness, the young age of the parents and the fact that Ricardo was the couple's first child. Beforehand, we recognised and valued intentionality, since the researcher's personal nature is involved when he or she takes a sensitive and understanding approach to human experiences that are so close to his or her existential reality (PETEAN, 2013).

To collect the empirical material, we used the In-Depth Interview, understood as a dialogue with intentionality (MINAYO, 2010), allowing the person to talk freely about their experience, with the researcher's questions being guided so as to gradually deepen certain narrative threads that emerge from the story (ARAÚJO et al., 2013), 2013); together, we used Observation, which enabled us to grasp the peculiar contexts of life and care, as well as the modes of expression that go beyond speech (ARAÚJO et al., 2013). These strategies were used to compose the Life Story of Ricardo's family, which we see as a privileged way of understanding the experiences of people and their families, as it involves someone 'telling' themselves to others and to themselves, and someone listening to this experience and colouring it, giving it relevance based on elements from their own experience (BELLATO; ARAÚJO, 2015).

So we held seven meetings between June 2015 and January 2016, four with Bruno present; and in the first two months we held weekly meetings with the family to bring the research team closer to their care experience. Of these, six were held at the family home, one at the baby's first birthday party and one at the maternity hospital, when Ricardo was hospitalised for the second time since his birth.

All the observation records, as well as the transcription of the narratives, made up the Research Diary (ARAÚJO et al, 2013), consisting of 230 pages typed in a Microsoft Word Document (docx) file, in Times New Roman font, size 12 and single spacing between the lines.

In order to understand the empirical material, we read all of it carefully and meticulously, trying to colour the excerpts in order to differentiate them according to their meanings. In an effort to interpret the family's experience, we tried to emphasise the elements that they themselves highlighted when telling and retelling moments that they considered important. In addition, the family has had access to the results of this study and has endorsed our "translation" of their experience, which serves as a "validator" that our efforts to understand, even if in a localised and approximate way, have been accepted by the family.

Through the intensive effort of approaching and distancing oneself from this material, various axes of meaning emerged, and this manuscript is the result of the axis

'Resignifications and perspectives of what is lived: the experience of having a child with the rare Schinzel-Giedion Syndrome'.

This axis of meaning was based on the analytical-synthesising drawing of the 'spiral of time', which highlighted the confluence of past, present and future in order to represent the resignifications of the time lived by Ricardo's family. This drawing, of a more interpretative nature, was reflected on in the research team's work meetings in order to emerge and converge, from this collective, subsidies for understanding the diverse and varied times of life and care.

According to Araújo and Lacerda (2008), drawing materialises mental images, constituting an interpretable sign as a representation of reality and shows that there is an intrinsic relationship between imagination and linguistic development.

This study respects and complies with the ethical prerogatives set out in Resolution 466/2012 (BRASIL, 2013), and the matrix research to which it is linked was approved under protocol 951.101/CEP-HUJM/2015. It is also important to emphasise that the family gave us the freedom to use the real names of the participants in this study. Therefore, with Bruno and Jéssica's consent, we have only used fictitious names for institutions and people mentioned by the couple.

RESULTS

Ricardo is a baby just over a year old, the first and only child of the young couple Jéssica and Bruno - both 24 - who are experiencing their first experiences of becoming parents and dealing with the repercussions of the rare syndrome that affects their son.

The hallmark of SSG is the shortening of the child's life expectancy and Ricardo's parents have learnt to deal with this situation in their daily lives in order to make the most of every shared moment. Thus, in their narratives, they make sense of the time they lived with Ricardo, giving rise to laborious reflections inspired by the poetics of Rubem Alves (1999, p.138), who tells us about the eternalisation of experiences that pass through the heart: "I felt *that time* is *just a thread. All the experiences of beauty and love that we've been through are threaded through it. What memory has loved remains eternal"*. In a similar way, it seems to us that the meaning of a child's life is taken as a gift, celebrated by their parents at every moment and in many ways that extend the time they live.

In this sense, the notion of 'temporality' provokes us to flex time in such a way as to supplant the linear and chronological idea of 'past-present-future', thinking of it as a confluence in which past and future overlap the present. Based on the family experience, the time lived was then imagistically presented in the drawing 'Spiral of the time lived in the family' (Figure 3), which guides the results of this study.

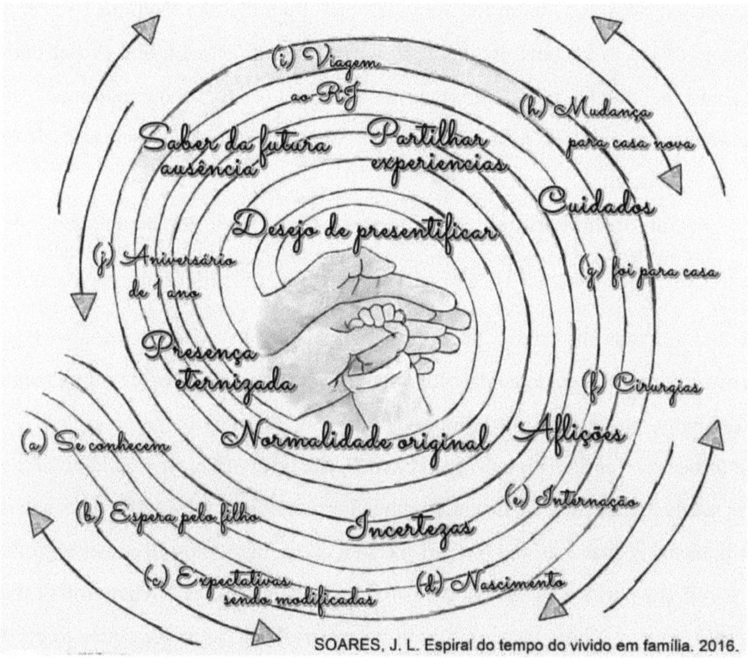

Figure 3 - Spiral of family time

In the centre of the drawing, we tried to represent Ricardo, his mother and his father by means of hands that support each other; around the hands and confluent with them are spiral lines that express the circularity of time, flanked on the outside by arrows that reinforce and characterise its movement, since the sense of experiential temporality is different in scope from chronological time, and is therefore not linear, through which we tried to show what happened in the family, in a present that is inexhaustible. Superimposed on the lines of the spiral, we distributed some words or narrative passages - signalled by lowercase letters of the alphabet from "a" to "j" - which, from the family's perspective, denote events that synthesise and are significant to what was experienced (Figure 3).

Expectations and new meanings for the young couple when starting a family: Ricardo is born!

Jéssica and Bruno met in high school (Fig. 3 - marking a), started dating when they were 16 and got married when they were 18. Six years later, they felt like having a baby and started planning for Jéssica to become pregnant; however, Ricardo came along earlier than planned. So the news that Jéssica was pregnant came as a kind of "foreboding surprise", as the couple had already foreseen the possibility. Bruno, overjoyed, took it upon himself to share the news with the rest of the family:

> I said to him "Bruno, wait for me to do the first ultrasound, right? to confirm it" [...] Ixi... when I saw he had already told everyone, I said "oh my God" [laughs] Then he was super happy, right mum? (Jéssica, mum).

In the joy that overtook the family, the young couple began to experience a new stage in their lives, permeated by expectations of becoming parents and, in this context, they made plans for the future baby, waiting anxiously for its arrival (Fig. 3 - mark b).

The sense of being a family is intensely marked by the birth of the first child, with the couple's attention gradually shifting to the child who is born. McGoldrick (2007) talks about this transition, emphasising that with the birth of the first child, the family becomes a group of three people, forming a permanent system that survives even if there is a separation or the death of one of the spouses. Thus, the family will never break up, as it continues to exist through the people who make it up.

The period of waiting for their son was quite intense for Jéssica and Bruno; however, during their antenatal appointments, they received information that their baby might be born with some alterations. This made the couple apprehensive and required them to readjust their plans to the new scenario that was unfolding; however, they didn't minimise the joy of the moments of waiting for Ricardo's arrival, but rather began the process of changing their future life plans 'for' and 'with' their son (Fig. 3 - marking c).

They therefore continued to gradually re-signify the experience of parenthood. In this respect, Fiamenghi Jr and Messa (2007) point out that parents often idealise a child in their minds, imagining the baby's sex, thinking about its school performance, career, sexual orientation, among other expectations.

With regard to their long-awaited first child, for Jéssica and Bruno, the event of the birth was transfigured in Ricardo's presence - the parents were expecting the most beautiful child, the healthiest, the cutest, the most everything! - However, their expectations were confronted by the marked changes in their baby and his prematurity, as he was born at 36 weeks gestation (Fig. 3 - mark d).

In this way, the changes warned about by the doctors left the realm of possibility and became present in the concreteness of life, and in an impactful way:

> We knew about a few problems during the pregnancy, but nothing major. Then when he was born, he was born with a lot of things! [...] there's a test that's done which is the karyotype, which looks at the DNA and so on, to see if there's any syndrome or not... And his was normal! And then, when he came out, he had the ear test, the foot test... Everything was altered, except the foot test (Bruno, father).

The first month of Ricardo's life took place in a Neonatal Intensive Care Unit (NICU) and Jéssica told us what it was like to experience the first few days with her son in hospital (Fig. 3, mark e) and her attempts to care for him maternally, as she had longed to do ever since she found out she was going to be a mum:

> [...] I wanted to hold him for a week and then I couldn't because he was still on oxygen and with a hood, so I couldn't hold him! Then I picked him up after a week when the psychologist saw that I was crying, wanting to hold him... Then she went and asked to be released. [...] After a week I started trying to breastfeed him, right? then... [Jéssica stops talking and continues to rub her son, then resumes speaking in a low tone of voice] then, it was one day that I tried, then the other day when I was going to take him anyway, to stay all day, he went back to the hood, then it was... I didn't pick him up for a few more days [speaks in a saddened tone]. (Jéssica, mum)

When her son was born, Jéssica hoped to take him home, introduce him to his room, bathe him and breastfeed him, and this is not what she and Bruno were able to do. On the contrary, the essentials, such as holding her son or feeding him his milk, were challenging and sometimes impossible, as well as being restricted to visits to the NICU, showing how much Jessica's expectations of being a mother were adjusted to the first demands that the SSG imposed on her baby, and also how little they were accepted by the professionals.

During this period, other events were considered quite distressing for Jéssica and Bruno - among them surgery due to a post-cesarean complication and the occurrence of anaemia (Fig. 3, mark f) - which they experienced while coming and going from hospital to visit their son. Especially for Jéssica, who was about to be hospitalised and was still worried about Ricardo in the NICU, this period was marked by her weak physical condition and also by loneliness, as Bruno, her constant companion, was unable to be there at this time:

> [...] then it was at the time of my other surgery that I had, right, because

> there was blood stuck and stuff, so I had to open up again... Then that day... I say it was the worst day ever! [pause] because it was the day he [Ricardo] went back to the hood and Bruno had travelled that day because he had an event out of town, and I was alone [sad speech] (Jéssica, mother).

When Ricardo was one month old, he was finally discharged from hospital and they were able to take him home (Fig. 3, mark g), but they carried with them uncertainties and anxieties - "[...] he wasn't *normal, he had a few problems, we didn't know what, right?"* (Bruno, father).

Perspectives on what is lived: learning to be a family alongside learning to care in Ricardo's original normality

On returning home, still without a diagnosis and with only the possibility of it being a rare syndrome, Jéssica and Bruno reorganised their lives and mobilised to meet the urgent and different needs that Ricardo presented over the course of the day: *"I stopped my life, her life and I ran every day. Every day I went for a check-up, a check-up. And then his little problems started to appear... and then we adapted* (Bruno, father). Day by day they also turned their lives more and more to Ricardo, 'enjoying their son', making many shared moments special - such as a simple walk: [...] At *least three times a week I take him* [Ricardo] *to my mum's* [...] *He likes to walk! He's a walker! He likes walking around other people's houses* [laughs] (Jéssica, mother).

The idea of 'enjoying the child' incorporates the notion of *carpe diem - a* Latin expression meaning "seize the day", in the sense of making the most of the 'now', appreciating the present of happiness. In this sense, living through Ricardo's normality includes differentiating his life span, shortened by the medical prognosis of degeneration that SSG imposes. This differentiation marks the son's life and, poignantly, his parents' experience with him, since it doesn't follow the natural course of farewells in life, in which the parents leave before the children.

In this study, while we consider the chronological time that accounts for 'life time' in the prognosis of SSG, we emphasise the subterranean dimension of 'lived time', an essential presence in human life, whose sense is expressed as 'temporality' because it is a subjectively perceived time. According to the authors, temporality spreads through the reverberations of experiences and, as such, emphasises how the past-present-future moves in spiral movements

(DOLINA; BELLATO; ARAÚJO, 2014).

In this way, Jéssica and Bruno continue to re-signify the experience of parenthood, of waiting for Ricardo to be born and throughout his first year, as a different being who lives a different time, offering him the best possible. The parents live 'with' and 'for' their son, in a present that expands in moments of sharing, while shaping their own future - for which they are also preparing in their lives today - as a valuable family legacy that they never want to break up.

In this direction, Ricardo's parents rethought the house they lived in, which didn't provide them with the comfort they needed and wasn't what they wanted to offer him. Jéssica made a point of emphasising how important the move to a new house was for the family (Fig. 3, mark h) and how it provided better conditions for looking after their son, reporting a careful concern to provide him with a welcoming place:

> [...] there [the old house] is a place where there's a lot of sewage, you know? There's agoutis, pigeons, stuff like that... So it's pretty unhealthy, you know?[...] I found a scorpion! [Yeah, here [the new house] there's space, you can go outside... Here, like Ricardo's trolley, I didn't even use it in the other house! It had been there for more than... Almost a year! Here I use it all the time!" (Jéssica, mum)

It seems to us, therefore, that the small house desired and won for Ricardo could be one of his family's happiness projects. According to the author (AYRES, 2007), happiness is a value sustained by concrete and fundamental experiences in human life, and its concreteness is related to the power to make us aware of what we experience as a Good. As such, this notion of happiness permeates family life and even shows itself through the care taken to tidy up the house, in the sense of it being a cosy place for Ricardo:

> Today I was able to take a closer look at the cosy living room of the house, and I noticed that it was very small [...] There were lots of family photos and also photos of the pregnancy. [...] Ricardo was sleeping peacefully on the sofa in the living room. Jessica carefully positioned him with his head and torso on a red cushion and his little legs stretched out on the sofa. It seemed an extremely comfortable position [...] Jéssica also took care to place a small fan in Ricardo's direction and the arm of the sofa acted as a shield so that the wind didn't hit the *boy* directly (Observation notes - 25.06.2015).

This cosiness offered to Ricardo brings us back to the idea of home as a place of emotional reference, beyond the possession of a physical space, which is an essential requirement for family life (PORTUGAL, 2014). It is therefore the most important place to live life, sharing the moments of happiness and suffering that make it up, as well as the intimacies of family life.

In this sense, Bachelard's (1993) reflection on what he calls the "nest house" is worth mentioning, alluding to our place of origin, where we return or dream of returning, just as the bird returns to the nest and the lamb returns to the fold. This sense "marks infinite daydreams, because human returns are made on the great rhythm of human life, a rhythm that crosses the years, that fights against all absences through the dream" (BACHELARD, 1993, p. 262).

It is also in this privileged place that things happen and take on their own close meaning for people, inscribed in the rhythms of routine, taking shape closer to habit than to the chronometer (BELLATO et al., 2011). It is in this daily context, taken as the world of the lived, that the family continues to provide care for Ricardo's life, such as feeding, making him sleep, bathing him, changing his nappies, among other cares that a baby needs, given his dependence on them to live at a young age. Undoubtedly essential, this care mixes with and adds to the care required by Ricardo's own normality due to the needs imposed by the rare syndrome. This 'blending' of care for life and Ricardo's original normality is described by Jéssica in minute detail in relation to giving her baby water and her own way of drinking it:

> I only give him water in a little syringe because this syringe is very small, right? he swallows it in the bottle, even with a thickener, which thickens it. [...] He's sucking on a dummy, so I take it and give it to him in the syringe. Then he drinks it and doesn't swallow it, but then you have to give it to him every few hours... (Jéssica, mum)

Such care for Ricardo's original normality is certainly labour-intensive and persevering, as Jéssica demonstrates when she tells us about breastfeeding her son:

> People, it was crazy! Because when he [Ricardo] got home, I was still... milking, saving to give to him and so on... And there was almost nothing coming out! Almost nothing was coming out! [...] I tried, I had that silicone nipple that you put in your breast, because my breast wasn't very big... The nipple, right? So he couldn't take it, he didn't recognise the nipple as something to suck on. So I put in that silicone nipple, then I put him [Ricardo] in... Sometimes he suckled a little but it was very little because he didn't have any strength in his mouth! The strength he really acquired was only a short time ago! Then I'd take out what he'd been sucking on, give him the powder I'd frozen, defrost it and give him the artificial one too! I gave him both! It was my milk and the pre-Nan that he took... Then the pre-Nan ended and we started with Nan!" (Jéssica, mum)

In the scene described, Ricardo's normal breastfeeding mobilised Jessica to look for ways to help him suckle because she understood that this is what a mother does - she breastfeeds her child with her milk; at the same time, she offers him additional nutritional support, meeting Ricardo's special need.

In order to highlight the minutiae of care that the family engenders, authors suggest the notion of a "myriad of care", which encompasses the different resources mobilised for each need of a loved one, so as to provide a lot of "small care", as well as means-actions so that other end-care can also be produced (SOUZA; ARAÚJO; BELLATO, 2016).

Jéssica and Bruno are learning to be parents by caring for Ricardo within the framework of normality. And to do so, they integrate care into their tasks that is even complex to carry out and would require specialised professional attention. Among these, they deal with the administration of medication through the gastrostomy - *because then you don't lose it, right?* (Jéssica, mum) - forms of stimulation for intestinal elimination - I *put the little laxative in the syringe, then I put the little probe in the syringe, I put a little oil on his little bum as well* (Jéssica, mum) - and nutritious preparations for feeding - *I beat everything after it's almost melted. Then I add more water and blend it, so it can go through the tube* (Jéssica, mum).

In this particularly unique context, Jessica has shown herself to be a very committed mother, even recognised by her husband:

> *Jéssica does everything... and his porridge is a lot of work and she spends a lot of time beating it and then sieves it and everything... It takes her ages to make it... It's very difficult* [laughs] *I don't know how to do any of these things, it's very difficult* [laughs]... *It's totally her medication, because I don't have any... She monitors, she knows, she schedules everything, so... I get lost sometimes. So, like... there's so much medicine... if I show you his medicine box, it's this big...* [shows the size with his hands] (Bruno, father)

Over time, Jéssica and Bruno have developed refined skills to recognise the signs that Ricardo shows when he's irritable or not feeling well, with the knowledge of experience shaping their own experience of caring for their son's life: [...] *before, when he got nervous, we'd massage him and he'd stop. Today, sometimes he calms down, but very little* [...] *You have to keep rubbing his hand* [he says, *rubbing* Ricardo's little hand] (Bruno, father).

Thus, we emphasise the existence of knowledge built on everyday experience and which supports family care, often incorporating specific health knowledge to the extent that the family perceives it to be understandable and possible to implement, making it useful in caring for the child (SCHNEIDER et al., 2015).

The parents take an 'attentive look' at Ricardo, so that when something happens that is not normal for him, they perceive it very acutely. As they refine this gaze, they continue to 'experiment' with ways of remedying his 'anxieties', while validating, on the basis of their responses, acts and attitudes of care that can help them or be effective in, to a certain extent, promoting his comfort and well-being.

Thus, it is in this context that Jessica and Bruno improve their ability to care for their son in his original normality, since they mobilise their care potential through an affectionate and very close relationship, in the very urgency of their needs and in the different situations that arise on a daily basis.

The way in which human potency expresses itself is unique and personalised, since each person can develop their potency in their own 'disposing themselves to', in an openness to the world, in which they offer something. In caring for life, this 'disposing oneself to' embodies involvement, readiness, attitudes and acts of care - which emphasises the relational dimension as its essential substance.

In this sense, authors (PETEAN; ARAÚJO; BELLATO, 2016) point out that the relationships between family members are fundamental in shaping care and, in addition to the needs that a health problem imposes, the ways in which family relationships are shaped are also elements that support care.

So, referring to the family in this study, the caring potentials need to be referred to the people of Jéssica - Bruno - Ricardo, regardless of how, in a situation, their potentials are transmuted from their latent form into support, help, support, sustenance and growth.

For the parents, the learning process is amplified and progresses with each need Ricardo presents, so they quickly learn to offer the best they have in caring acts and attitudes. To do this, they take into account their son's particularities, which have been and are learnt in the midst of a continuous, close and intimate relationship, mediated by the senses that emerge to perceive Ricardo, given that his ways of 'saying' have their own expressive subtlety.

> [...] Then... [turns his attention to his son and says affectionately] What's wrong Mum? [pauses his speech and looks intently at his son] He's having a spasm! [Noticing the discreet and continuous movements Ricardo is making with his arms. Jéssica remains for a few seconds without saying anything, just running her hands over her son's legs and arms]. (Jéssica, mum)

In this context, sharing experiences with other families experiencing similar situations has been a great help in supporting Ricardo's care. Jéssica and Bruno say it's even a way of learning to deal with the compromises resulting from the syndrome: "We don*'t know more or less what's going on, what's going to happen. We post everything in the group, and the people* *respond immediately [...] immediately... "* (Bruno, father). Of course, families experience their children's original normality by constituting knowledge from experience; this can be shared, even offering some practical answers to the problems that arise.

The group referred to by Bruno is called 'Schinzel-Giedion Syndrome' and is organised on a worldwide social network, in which families living with SSG participate. They try to exchange care experiences, tell about their children's achievements and post photos of them, in order to share their experiences with different families around the world.

In this way, the group becomes a kind of place where families can express the normality they experience with their children and recognise similarities between the children. This is a very encouraging and motivating possibility for parents to continue providing the best care for their children:

> [...] and then he took the exams, did a lot of things and so on... and without any good expectations, nothing... Nothing got better, everything got worse... And then we found out that all the other children were already using gastro, right? And we got round to doing it as soon as possible. So, the good thing about him is that... He was the youngest of the group [referring to the group of parents with children who have the same syndrome], so everything the family was already doing, was already happening, we were already running around and doing it as soon as possible because his life expectancy is two-three years, which is when children die, right?

On the other hand, when Ricardo's original normality is dealt with and accepted by his parents, there are the expectations of others who confront it, the most apparent point of which is the child's developmental pattern during the first year of life. A child is expected to start changing position, then sitting up and crawling, in order to prepare for the first steps. In a way, Bruno recognises this clash of expectations in his mother towards her son: *My mother, to this day, doesn't really believe that he's like that. She comes home every time, every day she asks: "Oh, he's not going to walk?"... "Oh, he's not going to talk to you, Grandma?"* (Bruno, father). Faced with their grandmother's wishes and often confronted by other views, they sometimes adopt strategies to make their expectations compatible with their son's original normality:

> *Sometimes I even lie about his age, right? Because his development is delayed. Then when I don't want to talk too much, I say: "No, he's seven months old"... Because if you say that he's going to be a year this big, all you'll have to do is swear at you, that you didn't feed him this, that and the other* (Jéssica, mum).

Living WITH and FOR your child in extending the 'gift' that celebrates life

We have learnt to categorise time chronologically, in seconds, minutes, hours, days, weeks, months, years, etc. It is in this "temporal form" that daily activities are circumscribed, each in its own chronological time, forming "overlapping layers", or "temporal extracts", because there must be a demarcated time to study, to work, to rest, to produce, among other human activities.

However, as we approach Jéssica and Bruno's experience with Ricardo, we realise another way of "living" in this time, which is expressed through experiential temporality. With their son, the parents live in a precious present that stretches towards tomorrows, which are sometimes uncertain: "So with *him like this* [...] we *don't know anything, it's everything... You don't know what tomorrow's going to be like, if he's going to sleep, if he's going to wake up* [...] *So every day is a surprise"* (Bruno, father).

In the face of Ricardo's original normality, every day is the 'best day' and every moment shared gains its valuable meaning in eternity.

> *Today he was smiling... well... Sometimes he smiles after a few spasms, right? Very slightly, then he has the spasms, then he smiles... Then today, at the counsellor's when she finished the session... he was half asleep, then when he woke up, at the end of the session, he smiled more and regained his face...* [laughs] *right Mum?* [speaks affectionately to Ricardo] (Jéssica, mother).

Faced with anguish and distress over the sombre medical prognosis of how long their child will live, parents try to make the most of the time they have for and with their child, even anticipating providing them with more appropriate care: *We can increase this expectation by doing everything as* soon *as possible...* Everything good for him, we'll do it as soon as possible. Like, the little children will have gastro at one year, a year and a bit... We've already done it when he was eight months old (Bruno, father).

Jéssica and Bruno monitor the existence of children with SSG in the world: Ricardo was the youngest, then last month 1 was born, so there are 2 [...] In my account here there are only 10 [alive]! [...] Yes, in the world of this group! In the group... (Jéssica, mum).

They were moved by two Brazilian families they met whose children had recently died, and they were overcome with fear for Ricardo:

> Then we found, we discovered two little children here in Brazil who had... one in Rio de Janeiro and the other in Bahia. [...] Then Mininho's father from Rio de Janeiro [...] I tried to contact him, sent him a message

> on the website and so on, and a few days later they replied. [...] Theirs had... died aged two years and four days, there in Rio... Two years and four days, right? And then we also managed to contact the family in Bahia. Then... he'd passed away a month before too... [she speaks very emotionally, like she's trying not to cry. She remains silent for a while and then resumes] So, it was the two we knew, right? [Silence] That was an even bigger shock! (Bruno, father)

> [...] but then there's the question that it's... the sad thing about this illness is that it seems [...] In my mind, it even seems that they are born with an expiry date [lowers tone of voice]. You know? because they pass away from silly things, you know? (Jéssica, mum)

Certainly, the possibility of near finitude echoes intensely in the hearts of the parents in a distressing and devastating feeling. However, this affliction did not end in itself, but rather pushed Jéssica and Bruno to mobilise their potential and develop new ones, using what they had at their disposal to create a driving force for perseverance, looking towards a horizon of hope. Hope lies in the very being of the child! And also in them, as the parents they are! So the affliction that causes concern can also 'cause care'; and it seems to us that this moves the young couple to look after their son. They use their affliction as a "forge" for hopeful perseverance.

With this persevering resistance, at the invitation of the family in Rio de Janeiro, Bruno and Jéssica decided to travel to meet them, taking their son with them (Fig. 3, mark i). This trip was a very special moment for the couple, as they got to know the family who had recently been through a similar situation to theirs, as well as tourist attractions and, above all, taking Ricardo for a walk:

> [...] Man, we used to take Ricardo to the beach in the buggy. You know? There's no such thing... I said: "Man, I don't know if he'll live, but at least he'll feel it, he'll feel the wind, he'll feel the air, he'll feel things too" (Bruno, father).

> People! He [Ricardo] went with me to Christ in a kangaroo... At Christ's he was uncomfortable, uncomfortable because he had colic, and it was very hot too... But so we went, where we went on the cable car there ixi! He was fine! He slept... Everything! (Jéssica, mum)

The couple reveal to us their horizon of hope, in which they aim against the 'expiry date' of the SSG, which circumscribes their son's life span. They believe in a time that needs to be well spent with him. Jéssica tells us that - 'when she sees Ricardo smiling, she stops doing what she's doing just to look at her son smile! - 'my son is going to see the sea' - and enjoyed the wind on his son's face on the beach he was enjoying... They therefore show us ways in which the precious present is stretched in the face of uncertain tomorrows.

We corroborate, the family embraces the needs of the child in a broad way, having a primary role in caring for life, in life and for life, from a perspective of the present, seeking to be well within the potentialities that present themselves in the here and now, not allowing the possibility of the closest finitude to be the deadly horizon that would annul this care (BELLATO et al., 2016).

It seems that Jéssica and Bruno don't turn their backs on the possibility of death - it's even a relevant concern, which can be seen in the 'follow-up' that Jéssica carries out on each child with SSG that she meets: I write down the parents' names, where they're from, when they were born and when they died. Because I can also see how many years they've lived, you know? (Jéssica, mum). However, it is life itself that they want to account for, enjoy and look at on the daily horizon.

As such, the future becoming is shown as a projection of what Jéssica and Bruno lived intensely 'with and for' their son. This becoming is also elaborated in the present with elements of the lived experience that can, in a way, perpetuate Ricardo's presence. So this desire for permanence (and the knowledge of his absence in the near future) takes place in the couple's daily life, embodied in their daily photographs and videos: And I film him every day, every hour... Every day I film, I take photos... there are more photos of him there... [Continues to show me the photos on his mobile phone] (Bruno, father).

The photographs, videos and also the online page that the couple maintain seem to us to have a meaning that goes beyond merely recording a moment in their lives, as they are ways of filling the spaces that the possible absence of their child will leave. In this future absence, there is a lot of presence in shared objects, rooms in the house, smells, flavours, memories...

Thus, the parents are concerned with keeping Ricardo's memory as a way of prolonging his stay, which is sure to be eternalised.

This desire for their son to remain in their lives is transfigured in the allegory of the angel, referenced by the couple in an original spiritual experience. In it, Jéssica describes how, when she became pregnant with Ricardo, she went to *a "little man who prayed, blessed, prayed, you know?".* He told her that "it was supposed *to be twins and then another pagan spirit didn't want him to be born".* So this man asked her: *do you want him to be born?"* To which she replied emphatically: *"Then I said, of course* [...] *of course I want my son to be born, right?"*. Then this gentleman told her about the child he was expecting: *"That he was a little angel sent by God, you know? That he was very special, that was one of the things he said"* (Jéssica, mother). From this short dialogue comes the allegory to which Jéssica refers to allude to Ricardo's presence in their lives. "Ricardo an angel sent by God" is the name given to the social network page they maintain, where they 'post' moments from Ricardo's life that they share more widely.

The celebration of Ricardo's life, with his victory over difficulties and also over death, takes place in many of the moments experienced by Jéssica and Bruno. One of these, which we were able to share, was his birthday party, which, as it took place in June, followed a country theme:

> *Right at the entrance, there was a wooden sign that read: Ricardo's Arraiá. At the door, a young man sat on a low chair with a small table in front of him, wearing a large straw hat and collecting tickets.* [...] *The whole place was decorated with colourful banners and there were some blue balloons in the pool. Ricardo looked very peaceful on his mum's lap, and I put my hand on his head and wished him a happy birthday.* [...] *From where I was sitting, I could see Jessica and her son. I noticed that there was a plastic cup on the* table containing Ricardo's diet and Jessica was using a syringe to feed him through the tube. [...] While I was there, at no time did Ricardo leave *his mother's* side (Observation notes - 20.06.2015).

Celebrating Ricardo's first birthday was very important to his parents, because the day their first and only child was born is an eternal milestone in their lives, so this date will always be remembered with warm feelings. So the celebration was important in terms of bringing family and friends together and being able to give thanks for the gift of life. In addition, it was a "different" day from the others, in which Jéssica and Bruno were able to experience, for the first time, the sensation of having a 'birthday' child.

CONCLUSIONS

The parents enjoy Ricardo's presence in an expanded present that is projected towards the future. Such an apprehension encourages us to think of the concept of time as a confluence in which the past and the future overlap the present, which is an inexhaustible source of the lived through which life gushes incessantly.

Thus, they experience a sense of happiness that is independent of what is conventionally considered to be complete well-being or perfect morphofunctional normality, notions that they relate to being healthy. Thus, they consider their child's original normality and, within it, the moments of illness and well-being that unfold over time.

The parents' experience shows us a way of perceiving Ricardo in his potential, which raises questions about the way we health professionals look at children who are born with some kind of 'difference', like Ricardo. In this sense, health professionals and services have a lot to learn from the lessons learnt by this family, which believes that

in the infinite potentiality of their son's becoming, where 'believing' has the meaning of 'knowing what is felt', and not just 'knowing what is known'. Therefore, they experience these potentialities as intensely viable and, given this, they mobilise themselves to help Ricardo move them forward and realise them within their original normality.

To this end, Jéssica and Bruno also put their caring powers into motion, modelling their care to the specific situations Ricardo presents and seeing how best to deal with them. In this way, they endeavour to offer Ricardo a family life that any child deserves. A life of care, concern and lots of love. All the preparation during pregnancy and the first year of his life show how much "the new normal" is present in family life. Not in imitation of the normality of an ordinary child, but the normality of the child's own needs, treated in a mature way by the parents as "the normality that is possible".

Parents' modelling of care for Ricardo is done in an integrative way, from the basic needs for his well-being, growth and development, to which are mixed and added those arising from the SSG. In this way, we grasp the notion of care that encompasses and integrates the needs of the beginning of human life, flowing and spreading through care during illness, care that considers the compromises and limitations of living, for which promptness and speed are essential.

BILIOGRAPHICAL REFERENCES

ALVES, R . Concerto para corpo e alma. 2 ed. Campinas - SP: Papirus, 1999.

ARAÚJO, C. C. M.; LACERDA, C. B. F. Examining children's drawing as a therapeutic resource for the language development of deaf children. Rev Soc Bras Fonoaudiol. v. 13, n 2, p. 186-92, 2008.

ARAÚJO, L. F. S. et al. Research diary and its potential in qualitative research. Brazilian Journal of Health Research, v. 15, n. 3, p. 53-61, 2013.

AYRES, J. R. C. M. A hermeneutical concept of health. Physis, v. 17, n. 1, p. 43-62, 2007.

BACHELARD, G. The poetics of space. 1 ed. São Paulo: Martins Fontes, 1993.

BELLATO, R.; ARAÚJO, L. F. S. Towards a comprehensive approach to the family care experience. Cienc Cuid Saude, v. 14, n. 3, p. 1394400, 2015.

BELLATO, R. et al. Family experience of care in chronic situations. Rev Esc Enferm USP, 2016. PRELO

BELLATO, R. et al. Mediation and mediators in the therapeutic itineraries of individuals and families in Mato Grosso. In: PINHEIRO, R.; MARTINS P. H. (Orgs.). Users, social networks, mediations and integrality in health. Rio de Janeiro: CEPESC/IMS-UERJ; Recife: UFPE, São Paulo: ABRASCO, 2011. p. 177-83.

BRAZIL. National Health Council. Approves regulatory standards for research involving human beings. Resolution no. 466, 12 December 2012. Lex: Federal Official Gazette. 2012 Jun.:01-52.

BRAZIL. Law No. 13.146, of 6 July 2015. Provides for the Statute of Persons with Disabilities. Federal Official Gazette, Brasília, 07 July 2015. Section 1, p. 02.

CARVALHO, E. et al. Schinzel-Giedion syndrome in two Brazilian patients: Report of a novel mutation in SETBP1 and literature review of the clinical features. American Journal of Medical Genetics. v. 167, n. 5, p. 1039-46, 2015.

CARTER, B.; MCGOLDRICK, M. Changes in the family life cycle: a framework for family therapy. 2. ed. Porto Alegre: Artmed, 2007. 511p.

DOLINA, J. V.; BELLATO, R.; ARAÚJO, L. F. S. Distinct temporalities in the breast cancer disease process. Rev. esc. enferm. USP, v. 48, n.2, p. 73-80, 2014.

DOLINA, J. V.; BELLATO, R.; ARAÚJO, L. F. S. Experience of young women and their families in becoming ill and dying from breast cancer. 2013. 118f. Dissertation (Master's in Nursing) - Postgraduate Programme in Nursing. Federal University of Mato Grosso, Faculty of Nursing, Cuiabá, 2013.

FIAMENGHI JR., G. A.; MESSA, A. A. Parents, children and disability: studies on family relationships. Psicol. cienc. prof. v.27, n.2, p. 236-45, 2007.

GONZÁLES, L. V. et al. Schinzel-Giedion syndrome: new mutation in SETBP1. An Pediatr (Barc), v. 82, n.1, p. 12-16, 2015.

MCGOLDRICK, M. Women and the family life cycle. In: CARTER, B.; MCGOLDRICK, M. (Orgs.). Changes in the family life cycle: a framework for family therapy. 2. ed. Porto Alegre: Artmed, 2007. ch. 2, p. 30-60.

MINAYO, M. C. S. O desafio do conhecimento: pesquisa qualitativa em saúde. 12 ed. São Paulo: Hucitec, 2010.

MINAYO, M. C. S.; GUERRIERO, I. C. Z. Reflexivity as the ethos of qualitative research. Ciênc. saúde coletiva. v. 19, n. 4, p. 1103-12, 2014.

PETEAN, E.; ARAÚJO, L. F. S.; BELLATO, R. Space-time dimension and the acts-attitudes of care in the family experience, 2016. J. res.: fundam. care. PRELO.

PETEAN, E. Substances of care in the family experience of illness: subsidies for professional care, 2013. 143f.
Dissertation (Master's in Nursing) - Postgraduate Course in Nursing, Faculty of Nursing, Federal University of Mato Grosso, Cuiabá, 2013.

PORTUGAL, S.; ALVES, J. P. Rare diseases and care: a look at social networks. In: IBEROAMERICAN CONGRESS ON RARE DISEASES, I, 2015, city. Proceedings. Coimbra: Centre for Social Studies - University of Coimbra, 2015. p. 34-40.

PORTUGAL, S. Famílias e Redes Sociais: Ligações fortes na produção de bem-estar. Editora Almedina: Coimbra, 2014.

SCHNEIDER, C. L. et al. Modelling family care in the chronic condition of adrenoleukodystrophy. Cienc Cuid Saude, v. 14, n. 2, p.1130- 38, 2015.

SOUZA, I. P.; ARAÚJO, L. F. S.; BELLATO, R. Care needs of young people experiencing a chronic situation due to concomitant diseases. Rev. Anna Nery, 2016. IN PRELO.

SOUZA, S. P. S. The repercussions of rheumatic fever and rheumatic heart disease on the lives of children and adolescents: the movement between feeling healthy and feeling ill. 2006. 238 f. Thesis (Doctorate) - Ribeirão Preto School of Nursing, University of São Paulo, Ribeirão Preto, 2006.

SOUZA, S. P. S; LIMA, R. A. G. Chronic condition and normality: towards the movement that expands the power to act and be happy. Rev Latino-am Enfermagem, v. 15, n. 1, p. 156-64, 2007.

FINAL CONSIDERATIONS

This study sought to stimulate important reflections, based on the many teachings that the family provides us with about their very personal way of caring for Ricardo "from, in and for life". We can see in the parents an acute and expanded sense of care that flows in different directions, spreading throughout their son's life, encompassing and integrating his needs in order to respond to them in the best possible way.

Thus, the urgency of integrating the many different types of care that Ricardo needs fills "a whole day" with the "little things" that are essential to his life. This is done by the family apart from a diagnosis that names the SSG, even before it is confirmed, since it relates to the 'knowledge of experience' that allows Jéssica and Bruno to "intuit" what might undermine the manifestations in their son's body. On the other hand, they see in the health professionals a diffuse perception, which takes Ricardo within the scope of his "expiry date" and produces, as a rule, feelings of disappointment and hopelessness in the family, given that there is so much to be done in terms of caring for the health of their son affected by the extremely rare and lethal syndrome.

In order to be reunited with hope, the family endeavours to get closer to other families who have experienced or will experience a similar situation, learning and teaching very personal ways of caring for their most precious possession - their child's life - in its own normality and in the flow of time that is possible. Therefore, the modelling of care by parents is done in an integrative way, encompassing and combining the needs at the beginning of human life, from the basic ones for its well-being, growth and development, to those determined by the SSG, considering the compromises and limitations 'of' and 'in' living, for which promptness and speed are essential.

In this sense, Jéssica and Bruno make an intense effort to find support of different kinds and in different places to help them provide the best care. However, they are sometimes faced with partial and fragmented responses from health professionals and services, who find it difficult to meet Ricardo's ever-expanding and renewed needs. It is therefore necessary to reflect on this rapid chronological time that shortens the possibilities 'in' and 'of' life, in order to use it efficiently and effectively to meet the very specific needs imposed by the HGS. Services and professionals need to do more than offer answers to specific health problems, they need to be able to support families in order to help them with the care they are so minutely shaping.

What the parents experienced showed temporalities scaled by different situations that had little to do with their chronological conception. We observed that the different temporalities experienced by Jéssica, Bruno and Ricardo intertwine over time towards a doomed destiny, and that is also why what they experienced was shaped into an extension of the 'present' that celebrates life and projects itself towards the near future, which is possible for Ricardo. This reflection encourages us to think of time as a confluence in which past and future overlap the present, the latter being an inexhaustible source of the lived through which life gushes incessantly.

The resolution capacity of services and professionals is of paramount importance and needs to be rethought in order to weigh up the protocol times in the field of health in relation to the different temporalities of each person's life. In Ricardo's situation, and that of so many other children with other conditions that limit their lives temporally, the exiguity and unpredictability of this time 'of and in' life prompts reflections on how services have managed to support families, taking into account the very particular needs they experience.

Due to the limitations of the focus of this study, other dimensions of the family's experience of caring for their child with a rare syndrome were not explored here. However, those dimensions that we have been able to address here give rise to important reflections and also concern the limited resolutiveness of health services, such as the multiple costs that the family incurs in order to provide the best care for their child and which remain, as a rule, in the order of the barely visible, be they material, social, emotional, psychological, among others, that come from caring. We would also point out that the research approach we took in this study proved to be very coherent and fruitful, making it possible to highlight sensitive images of everyday family care, since it favoured dialogue between cognition, imagination and sensitivity, traversing the milieus of a contemporary science that integrates the multiplicity of human knowledge.

Finally, the construction of this study has been a gift of life for the master's student who, in the context of mutual affections, has learnt great lessons from Jéssica, Bruno and Ricardo about happiness and hope, not in the sense of "waiting", but of "hoping", which implies continuous and encouraging effort and movement to always offer the best we can in the most diverse situations that arise throughout human life.

BIBLIOGRAPHICAL REFERENCES

ALBANO, L. M. J. et al. Hydronephrosis in schinzel-giedion Syndrome: an important clue for the diagnosis. Rev. Hosp. Clin. Fac. Med. S. Paulo, v. 59, n. 2, p, 89-92, 2004.

ALMEIDA, K. B. B.; ARAÚJO, L. F. S.; BELLATO, R. Family care in the experience of a young person's chronic illness. Rev Min Enferm. v. 18, n. 3, p.724-32, 2014.

ALVES, R. Concerto para corpo e alma. 2 ed. Campinas - SP: Papirus, 1999.

ALVES, J. P. Ethnographer bringing home: notes on the strangeness of looking at the other in their home. Oficina do CES, n. 426, 2015. Available at: <http://www.ces.uc.pt/publicacoes/oficina/ficheiros/12645_Oficina_do_CE S_426.pdf>. Accessed on: 20 September 2015.

ARAÚJO, C. C. M.; LACERDA, C. B. F. Examining children's drawing as a therapeutic resource for the language development of deaf children. Rev Soc Bras Fonoaudiol. v. 13, n 2, p. 186-92, 2008.

ARAÚJO, L. F. S. et al. Research diary and its potential in qualitative research. Brazilian Journal of Health Research, v. 15, n. 3, p. 53-61, 2013.
AYRES, J. R. C. M. A hermeneutical concept of health. Physis, v. 17, n. 1, p. 43-62, 2007.

AYRES, J. R. C. M. et al. The concept of Vulnerability and Health Practices: new perspectives and challenges. In: CZERESINA, D.; FREITAS, C. M. (Org). Health Promotion: concepts, reflections, trends. Rio de Janeiro: Fiocruz, 2003. 176 p. 5.

BACHELARD, G. The poetics of space. 1 ed. São Paulo: Martins Fontes, 1993.

BACHELARD, G. A dialética da duração. 2 ed. São Paulo: Ática; 1994.

BELLATO, R. The sick person's experience of hospitalisation. 2001.
209f. Thesis (Doctorate) - Ribeirão Preto School of Nursing, University of São Paulo, Ribeirão Preto, 2001.

BELLATO, R. et al. Focal Life History and its potential in health and nursing research. Electronic Rev. Enf., v.10, n.3, p. 849-56, 2008.

BELLATO, R. et al. Mediation and mediators in the therapeutic itineraries of individuals and families in Mato Grosso. In: PINHEIRO, R.; MARTINS P. H. (Orgs.). Users, social networks, mediations and integrality in health. Rio de Janeiro: CEPESC/IMS-UERJ; Recife: UFPE, São Paulo: ABRASCO, 2011. p. 177-83.

BELLATO, R.; ARAÚJO, L. F. S. Towards a comprehensive approach to the family care experience. Cienc Cuid Saude, v. 14, n. 3, p. 1394400, 2015.

BELLATO, R. et al. Family experience of care in chronic situations. Rev Esc Enferm USP, 2016. PRELO

BRAZIL. National Health Council. Approves regulatory standards for research involving human beings. Resolution no. 466, 12 December 2012. Lex: Federal Official Gazette. 2012 Jun.:01-52.

BRAZIL. Law No. 13.146, of 6 July 2015. Provides for the Statute of Persons with Disabilities. Federal Official Gazette, Brasília, 07 July 2015. Section 1, p. 02.

BRAZIL. Ministry of Health. Ordinance No. 199 of 30 January 2014. Approves the National Policy for Comprehensive Care for People with Rare Diseases. Federal Official Gazette. 2014.

CARVALHO, E. et al. Schinzel-Giedion syndrome in two Brazilian patients: Report of a novel mutation in SETBP1 and literature review of the clinical features. American Journal of Medical Genetics. v. 167, n. 5, p. 1039-46. 2015.

CARTER, B.; MCGOLDRICK, M. Changes in the family life cycle: a framework for family therapy. 2. ed. Porto Alegre: Artmed, 2007. 511p.

CASTELLANOS, M. E. P. Narrative in qualitative health research. Ciênc. saúde coletiva, v 19, n. 4, p.1065-76, 2014.

CORAZZA, S. M. Labyrinths of research, before the bolts. In: COSTA, M. V. Caminhos investigativos I. 3. ed. Rio de Janeiro: Lamparina editora, 2007. chap. 5, p. 103-28.

COSTA, A. L. R. C. et al. The journey in the construction of therapeutic itineraries for families and networks for care. In: PINHEIRO, R.; MARTINS P. H. (Org.). Avaliação em saúde na perspectiva do usuário: abordagem multicêntrica. Recife: UFPE, Rio de Janeiro: CEPESC/IMS- UERJ/ABRASCO, 2009. p. 195-202.

DOLINA, J. V.; BELLATO, R.; ARAÚJO, L. F. S. Distinct temporalities in the breast cancer disease process. Rev. esc. enferm. USP, v. 48, n.2, p. 73-80, 2014.

DOLINA, J. V.; BELLATO, R.; ARAÚJO, L. F. S. Experience of young women and their families in becoming ill and dying from breast cancer. 2013. 118f. Dissertation (Master's in Nursing) - Postgraduate Programme in Nursing. Federal University of Mato Grosso, Faculty of Nursing, Cuiabá, 2013.

FIAMENGHI JR., G. A.; MESSA, A. A. Parents, children and disability: studies on family relationships. Psicol. cienc. prof. v.27, n.2, p. 236-45, 2007.

FIOVARANTI, C. The cobblestone path of rare diseases. Revista Pesquisa FAPESP, São Paulo, Aug. 2014. Available at: <http://revistapesquisa.fapesp.br/2014/08/21/o-caminho-de-pedras-das- doencas-raras/>. Accessed on: 10 September 2015.

GALEANO, E. The Book of Hugs. Translated by Eric Nepomuceno. 9. ed Porto Alegre: L&PM, 2002. 270p.

GERHARDT, T. E. et al. Sensitive criteria for measuring the repercussions of professional care on the lives of individuals, families and communities. In: PINHEIRO, R.; SILVA JUNIOR, A. G. (Org.). Por uma sociedade cuidadora. 1. ed. Rio de Janeiro: CEPESC/IMS-UERJ/ABRASCO, 2010. chap. XX, p. 293-306.

GONZÁLES, L. V. et al. Schinzel-Giedion syndrome: new mutation in SETBP1. An Pediatr (Barc), v. 82, n.1, p. 12-16, 2015.

GUTIERREZ, D. M. D.; MINAYO, M. C. S. Production of knowledge on health care within the family. Ciência e Saúde Coletiva, v. 15, sup. 1, p. 1497-508, 2010.

HOISCHEN, A. et al. De novo mutations of SETBP1 cause Schinzel- Giedion syndrome. Nature Genetics, v. 42, n. 6, p. 483-85, 2010.

LEHMAN, A. M. et al. Schinzel-Giedion syndrome: Report of splenopancreatic fusion and proposed diagnostic criteria. Am J Med Genet, v. 146A, n. 10, p. 1299-306, 2008.

MAFFESOLI, M. The fertile soil of everyday life. FAMECOS Magazine, n. 36, p. 5-9, 2008.

MARTINS, A. J. et al. The conception of family and religiosity present in the discourses produced by medical professionals about children with genetic diseases. Ciência e Saúde Coletiva, v. 17, n. 2, p. 545-53, 2012.

MCGOLDRICK, M. Women and the family life cycle. In: CARTER, B.; MCGOLDRICK, M. (Orgs.). Changes in the family life cycle: a framework for family therapy. 2. ed. Porto Alegre: Artmed, 2007. ch. 2, p. 30-60.

MENDES, E. V. The care of chronic conditions in primary health care: the imperative of consolidating the family health strategy. Brasília: Pan American Health Organisation, 2012. 512 p.

MINAYO, M. C. S. O desafio do conhecimento: pesquisa qualitativa em saúde. 12 ed. São Paulo: Hucitec, 2010.

MINAYO, M. C. S.; GUERRIERO, I. C. Z. Reflexivity as the ethos of qualitative research. Ciênc. saúde coletiva. v. 19, n. 4, p. 1103-12, 2014.

MORIN, E. Where is the world going? Translation by Francisco Morás. 2 ed. Rio de Janeiro: vozes, 2010.

MUFATO, L. F. et al. (Re) organisation in family daily life due to the repercussions of chronic cancer. Ciência Cuidado e Saúde, v. 11, n. 1, p. 89-97, 2012.

MUSQUIM, C. A. Experience of care by men in the family experience of chronic illness. 2013. 141 f. Dissertation (Master's in

Nursing) - Postgraduate Course in Nursing. Federal University of Mato Grosso, Faculty of Nursing, Cuiabá, 2013.

OLIVEIRA, R. G; MARCON, S. S. Working with families in the Family Health Programme: the practice of nurses in Maringá-Paraná. Rev Esc Enferm USP. v. 41, n. 1, p. 65-72, 2007.

OLIVEIRA, R. F. Existence: St Augustine and his reflection on time. Science & Life Portal. Available at: <http://filosofiacienciaevida.uol.com.br/ESFI/Edicoes/33/artigo130300- 1.asp>. Accessed on: 26 August 2015.

UNITED NATIONS ORGANISATION. Universal Declaration of Human Rights, adopted on 10 December 1948.

WORLD HEALTH ORGANISATION. Innovative care for chronic conditions: structural components for action. World report. Brasilia: DF, 2002.

OVIEDO, R. A. M.; CZERESNIA, D. The concept of vulnerability and its biosocial character. Interface, v. 19, n. 53, p. 237-49, 2014.

PETEAN, E.; ARAÚJO, L. F. S.; BELLATO, R. Space-time dimension and the acts-attitudes of care in the family experience, 2016. J. res.: fundam. care. PRELO.

PETEAN, E. Substances of care in the family experience of illness: subsidies for professional care, 2013. 143f.
Dissertation (Master's in Nursing) - Postgraduate Course in Nursing, Faculty of Nursing, Federal University of Mato Grosso, Cuiabá, 2013.

PORTUGAL, S.; ALVES, J. P. Rare diseases and care: a look at social networks. In: IBEROAMERICAN CONGRESS ON RARE DISEASES, I, 2015, city. Proceedings. Coimbra: Centre for Social Studies - University of Coimbra, 2015. p. 34-40.

PORTUGAL, S. Famílias e Redes Sociais: Ligações fortes na produção de bem-estar. Editora Almedina: Coimbra, 2014.

SILVA, A. H. Experience of illness and care of a family living with chronic sickle cell anaemia of two

teenagers, 2012. 141 f. Dissertation (Master's in Nursing) - Postgraduate Course in Nursing. Federal University of Mato Grosso, Faculty of Nursing, Cuiabá, 2012.

SILVA, A. H.; BELLATO, R.; ARAÚJO, L. F. S. Daily life of the family experiencing the chronic condition of sickle cell anaemia. Revista Eletrônica de Enfermagem, v. 15, n. 2, p. 437-436, 2013.

SÁNCHEZ, A. I. M.; BERTOLOZZI, M. R. Can the vulnerability concept support the construction of knowledge in collective health care? Ciência & Saúde Coletiva, v. 12, n. 2, p. 319-24, 2007.

SCHNEIDER, C. L. et al. Modelling family care in the chronic condition of adrenoleukodystrophy. Cienc Cuid Saude, v. 14, n. 2, p.1130- 38, 2015.

SOUZA, I. P.; ARAÚJO, L. F. S.; BELLATO, R. Care needs of young people experiencing a chronic situation due to concomitant diseases. Rev. Anna Nery, 2016. IN PRELO.

SOARES, J. L. et al. Considerations about the health tie in the trajectory of search for elderly and the family care. J. res.: fundam. care, v. 5, n. 4, p. 583-90, 2013a.

SOARES, J. L. et al. Weaving the health bond in the family situation of illness. Rev. Interface. v. 21, n. 60, 2017. IN PRELO.

SOARES, J. L. et al. Demand for surgeries mediated by the judiciary: considerations on the right to health. Revista Baiana de Saúde Pública, v. 35, n. 4, p. 898-910, 2011.

SOUZA, I. P.; ARAÚJO, L. F. S.; BELLATO, R. Care needs of young people experiencing a chronic situation due to concomitant diseases. Rev. Anna Nery, 2016. IN PRELO.

SOUZA, S. P. S. The repercussions of rheumatic fever and rheumatic heart disease on the lives of children and adolescents: the movement between feeling healthy and feeling ill. 2006. 238 f. Thesis (Doctorate) - Ribeirão Preto School of Nursing, University of São Paulo, Ribeirão Preto, 2006.

SOUZA, S. P. S; LIMA, R. A. G. Chronic condition and normality: towards the movement that expands the power to act and be happy. Rev Latino-am Enfermagem, v. 15, n. 1, p. 156-64, 2007.

STARFIELD, B. Primary care - Balancing health needs, services and technology. Brasília: UNESCO, Ministry of Health, 2002. 726p. Available at: < http://bvsms.saude.gov.br/bvs/publicacoes/atencao_primaria_p1.pdf>. Accessed on: 7 September 2015.

THOMPSON, E. P. Time, labour discipline and industrial capitalism. In: Common Customs: Studies in Popular Culture traditional. 1 ed. São Paulo: Cia das Letras. 1998. p. 1267-304.

VAN VELSEN, J. Situational analysis and the detailed case study method. In: FELDMAN-BIANCO, Bela (Org.). Anthropology of contemporary societies: methods. 2ª ed. São Paulo: UNESP, 2010.

FEDERAL UNIVERSITY OF MATO GROSSO. Subsidies for modelling the care of families in situations of vulnerability - Research Project, institutional registration n°131/CAP/2014. 2015. Mato Grosso, 2014. 10p.

APPENDICES

Appendix I - Research Diary Instrument

FEDERAL UNIVERSITY OF MATO GROSSO

FACULTY OF NURSING

NURSING HEALTH AND CITIZENSHIP RESEARCH GROUP

MATRIX RESEARCH: **AIDS FOR MODELLING CARE FOR FAMILIES IN SITUATIONS OF VULNERABILITY**

RESEARCH DIARY

FAMILY PARTICIPANT

WORK CELL

CUIABÁ-MT

START: /END: /

(month / year)

RESEARCH DIARY

MATRIX RESEARCH: **SUPPORT FOR MODELLING CARE FOR FAMILIES IN SITUATIONS OF VULNERABILITY**

I - GENERAL GUIDELINES FOR COMPOSING THE RESEARCH DIARY[1]

The Research Diary is intended for recording research, consisting of an **observation** report (A), a transcript of each **interview** meeting (B) and **elaborations by the researcher/work cell/research group** (C) related to the methodological path and the interpretative work on the *corpus* analysing the family situation under study.

It is a unique instrument for each family situation studied and in it, each participating researcher writes down elements related to what they have heard, noticed, observed and experienced.

The information collected during fieldwork should be filled in immediately after each field entry.

The notes below in A, B and C are intended to highlight important elements to be taken into account when composing this diary.

A - OBSERVATION REPORT

PEOPLE: people present, people's appearance, interactions during meetings in relation to family members and the researcher(s), styles and ways of saying themselves and the other, snippets of conversations, silences, body language (posture and emotional responses, expressions, discomfort, looks, speech and tone of voice, gestures).
PLACES: description of the environment and its context, objects that have caught your eye, their arrangement, the use and occupation of the spaces by the people in the family, scenes from everyday life that take place during the interviews.
ACHIEVEMENTS IN RESEARCH: how the search for the participating family took place, the preparation of the research team for entering the field, the first contact with the family, how the situations during the fieldwork were experienced by each member of the research team, including the perception of their welcome by the interviewee/family, interruptions in the fieldwork, embarrassing situations that occurred during the meeting, problems with the equipment used in the field, how the family said goodbye to leave the field.

B - INTERVIEW TRANSCRIPT

WHEN TO TRANSCRIBE: the recorded interview should be transcribed immediately after each meeting.
HOW TO TRANSCRIBE: use a fictitious name for each participant in the study, in order to preserve their identity, as well as that of the institutions and people they mention; name the speech of each deponent and each interviewer when transcribing the narratives: the transcription record should be as faithful as possible to the spoken language and. The transcription record should be as faithful as possible to the spoken language and, in it, to each person's way of saying things; point out the different intonations of voice, as well as silences and other modes of expression; relate the narrative to the context in which it takes place, whenever important. To emphasise the nuances of speech, use grammatical resources to transcribe the narratives, accompanied by subtitles that allow them to be understood. For example, based on Almeida's dissertation (2012)

- Font in italics: size 12 for passages where the voice varies little in intensity; size 10 for a slightly lower voice, but understandable; size 08 for very low speech, difficult to understand, requiring effort to understand what is being said; size 14 for a stronger voice throughout the speech; size 16 for very loud speech.
- Speech between two dashes, bolded and underlined: represents the speech of one participant that crosses the speech of another who is reporting some fact, so that both speeches are united within a passage. Also used for expressions of agreement or negation that do not interrupt the main speech.

C - ELABORATIONS BY THE RESEARCHER / WORK CELL / RESEARCH GROUP

INSIGHTS OF THE RESEARCHER: the insiglits and impressions of the researcher(s) regarding the information gathered by observation and interview should be highlighted in the "FIRST READING AND PRE-ANALYSIS" column, by means of: key words, topics, focus, phrases used by the interviewee, and which seem to give a "tone" to their narrative.
QUESTIONS AND LEARNINGS: what the researcher learnt from the meeting, as well as their difficulties, personal challenges, learnings as a researcher and ideas for future meetings.
DISCUSSIONS SUBMITTED BY THE WORKING CELL / RESEARCH GROUP: composed of preliminary ideas, strategies and theoretical and methodological reflections throughout the research work generated in the discussions held after each meeting with the participating family by the working cell and also by the research group; recorded in the form of a summary, diagram, drawing, photos and others, in order to emerge themes that need to be explored in depth in subsequent meetings with the family, as well as to draw up "the state of the art of research" relating to the family.

II - NAMES OF RESEARCH TEAM MEMBERS

Postgraduate student:

Undergraduate student:

IH BREÁ~E REPORT OF THE SITUATION MVENC 1 EXPERIENCED BY THE FAMILY

IV - COMPOSITION OF THE PARTICIPATING FAMILY AND ITS MEMBERS

NAME	DEGREE OF KINSHIP	AGE	SCHOOLING	PROFESSION[1] OCCUPATION	RELIGION	PROBLEM OF HEALTH/DISEASE	REMARKS

OBS - This table can be filled in during the fieldwork and it is important that it is complete, with all family members, regardless of whether they live in the same house or not.

V - HEALTH AND OTHER INSTITUTIONS USED BY THE FAMILY

NAME OF INSTITUTION	RELATIONSHIP BETWEEN THE FAMILY AND THE INSTITUTION AND VICE VERSA	FREQUENCY OF USE OF THE INSTITUTION	SUPPORT PROVIDED	PERSON FROM THE INSTITUTION REFERRED TO BY THE FAMILY (LINK)

M DATES F. DURATION OF LABOUR DF. FIELD:

DATE \ DF EACH INTERVIEW DATE	DURATION OF THE INTERVIEW MEETING	members of the eqtpe researcher	FAMILY MEMBERS AT THE MEETING	PEOPLE INTERVIEWED	REMARKS

MI ANALYSING DRAWINGS PRODUCED IN THE RESEARCH (DIAGRAM, GENOGRAM, NETWORKS FOR CARE, TRAJECTORIES. MDA LINE. ETC):

MII RESEARCH PRODUCTS FOR THE PERIOD / TO /

BIBLIOGRAPHICAL REFERENCES

ALMEIDA. K. B. B. Experience of chronic illness due to concomitant conditions and care in the lives of young people and their families. 2012. 155 f. Dissertation (Master's) - Faculty of Nursing. Federal University of Mato Grosso. Cuiabá. 2012.

ARAÚJO. L. F. S.: DOLINA. J.; PETEAN. E.; MUSQUIM. C. A.; BELLATO. R.; LUCIETTO. G C. Research diary and its potential in qualitative health research. Rev. **Bras. Pesq. Saúde,** v. 15. n. 3. p. 53-61. jul-sept.. 2013.

<table>
<tr><td colspan="2">REGISTRATION INSTRUMENT N*</td></tr>
<tr><td colspan="2">NAME OF THE RESEARCHERS AT THE INTERVIEW MEETING:
DATE OF FIELDWORK:
START: END:
MEETING TIME:
RECORDING TIME OF THE MEETING:
LOCATION:
ADDRESS:
CITY: ' STATE:
PHONE RARA CONTACT:
FAMILY MEMBERS PRESENT AT THE MEETING:
NAME OF INTERVIEWEE(S):
* fictitious name</td></tr>
<tr><td colspan="2">A- OBSERVATION REPORT
Carried out by (identification of researcher):</td></tr>
<tr><td>use as many lines as necessary</td><td>FIRST READING AND PRE-ANALYSIS</td></tr>
<tr><td colspan="2">B - TRANSCRIPT OF INTERVIEW Carried out by (identification of researcher):</td></tr>
<tr><td>use as many lines as necessary</td><td>FIRST READING AND PRE-ANALYSIS</td></tr>
<tr><td colspan="2">C THE RESEARCHER'S ELABORATIONS WORK CELL WORK GROUP RESEARCH</td></tr>
</table>

Carried out by (identification of researcher):
use as many lines as necessary

Appendix II - Addendum to the Informed Consent Form

FEDERAL UNIVERSITY OF MATO GROSSO SCHOOL OF NURSING ADDENDUM TO THE INFORMED CONSENT FORM

You have been invited to take part, as a volunteer, in the research **"Subsidies for modelling care for families in situations of vulnerability"** and, after being informed about it, you have agreed to take part in the study conducted by Master **Juliana de Lima Soares** by signing the Free and Informed Consent Form. Through this consent form, you have been assured that the data relating to you will be kept confidential and that your participation in the research will be kept secret, including its dissemination, by means of anonymity.

At the time of the interviews, as a participant in the research, you expressed **your** wish for **your real name and that of your child to be declared in the study,** which **would** result in your identification and therefore a breach of the anonymity guaranteed to you.

Considering this desire, this **Addendum to the Free and Informed Consent Form** aims to ensure that you give us your Free and Informed Consent for your name and that of your child, full name or first name, to be disclosed in the studies produced from the interviews carried out, both in the academic environment and in scientific publications in the health and related fields.

The purpose of this addendum is also to reaffirm **the ethical precaution of fidelity to the information you provide,** by guaranteeing knowledge of the content of the results in which you and/or your child are named; and your manifestation accepting their disclosure and/or publication.

You will receive a copy of this addendum with my name, telephone number and address, as the researcher responsible for this research, so that you can locate me at any time. My name is Laura Filomena Santos de Araújo, I am a lecturer at the Faculty of Nursing at the Federal University of Mato Grosso. My institutional address is Av. Fernando Corrêa da Costa, n° 2367 - Bairro Boa Esperança, Cuiabá - MT - CEP; 78060-900. My institutional contact telephone number is (65) 3615-8805 and my e-mail address is laurafill@yahoo.coin.br.

If you would like to contact the Research Ethics Committee itself, you can get in touch with the committee's coordinator, Shirley Ferreira Pereira, at Rua Luís Philippe Pereira Leite, S/N - Alvorada - Cuiabá-MT - CEP: 78048-902 or by calling the institutional contact number (65) 3615-7254.

Considering the above data, I **CONFIRM** that I have been informed in writing and verbally of the content of this addendum to the Informed Consent Form.

I (name of participant).. ....,...., ...,.... ....
age:....... sex:Place ....of birth: .... ID card holder
N°:......................authorisethat my real name and that of my son be published in the studies produced on the basis of the interviews carried out, both in academic circles and in scientific publications in the field of health and the like.

Signature of participant (or guardian, if a minor):...

Signature of principal investigator:...

Witness*: ....
* A witness is only required if the participant is unable to sign the form for any reason.

Date (City of/day month and year) Cuiabá , 2016.

ANNEXES

Annex I - Informed Consent Form

FEDERAL UNIVERSITY OF MATO GROSSO
FACULTY OF NURSING
FREE AND INFORMED CONSENT FORM

You are being invited to take part, as a volunteer, in the study "Subsidies for modelling care for families in situations of vulnerability" and you may withdraw your consent at any time during the study. Once you have been informed about the following information and agree to take part in the study, please sign this document, which is in two copies, one of which is yours and the other is for the researcher responsible. If you do not wish to take part in the study, you will not be harmed in any way in your relationship with the researcher or the institution where you receive care. If you have any questions, you can contact the Research Ethics Committee of the Júlio Miiller University Hospital - UFMT - on (65) 36157254.

The aim of this study is to understand the care potential of families in situations of vulnerability in order to support care modelling. Your participation in this research will consist of an interview (recorded and/or filmed) and observation focusing on your family's experience of care and illness, how you care for yourselves and are cared for in terms of your health needs, and also the help and support you receive from health professionals in the face of the difficulties you face in this experience. The interview will take place at a place and time of your choice, and after the first interview we will arrange the next ones as necessary.

With regard to the benefits of your participation in the research, the results of the study are important for the training of health professionals, in order to improve professional care for families. This study can also bring subjective gains for you, in terms of listening to your experience, as well as the respectful relationship throughout our meetings. You may withdraw from the interview at any time.

Your interview will form part of a research database that can be used for future studies. In this database, managed by the coordinator of this research, your complete anonymity is guaranteed, as well as respect for your wishes to have your information in it, and to remain there or not as long as it is in your interest.

We guarantee the accuracy of the information you give us. Your personal data will be kept confidential and we guarantee the secrecy of your participation throughout the research, including its dissemination. As such, we will maintain your complete anonymity and no-one other than the researchers will have access to your name as a participant in this research.

You will receive a copy of this form with my name, telephone number and address, as the researcher responsible for this research, so that you can locate me at any time. My name is Lauta Filomena Santos de Araújo, I am a lecturer at the Faculty of Nursing at the Federal University of Mato Grosso, my institutional contact telephone number is (65) 3615-8805 and my e-mail address is laurafilliirvahoo.com.br.

Considering the above data. I CONFIRM that I have been informed in writing and verbally of the objectives of this research.

I (name of participant)..,
age............. :sex: ....Place of .... birth: ID card holder
N°:.............................I declare that I have understood the objectives, risks and benefits of my participation in research and agree to participate.

Signature of participant (or guardian, if a minor): ....

Signature of principal investigator: ....

Witness*................................ .. ..
* A witness is only required if the participant is unable to sign the document for some reason.

Date (City'day month and year)of 20______________________________

Annex II - Ethics Approval Report

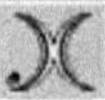

HOSPITAL UNIVERSITÁRIO JÚLIO MULLER- UNIVERSIDADE FEDERAL DE

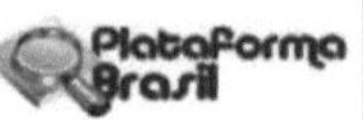

PARECER CONSUBSTANCIADO DO CEP

DADOS DO PROJETO DE PESQUISA

Título da Pesquisa: SUBSÍDIOS PARA A MODELAGEM DO CUIDADO DE FAMÍLIAS EM SITUAÇÕES DE VULNERABILIDADE

Pesquisador: Laura Filomena Santos de Araújo

Área Temática:

Versão: 2

CAAE: 39285114.8.0000.5541

Instituição Proponente: Faculdade de Enfermagem - Cuiabá - UFMT

Patrocinador Principal: Financiamento Próprio

DADOS DO PARECER

Número do Parecer: 951.101

Data da Relatoria: 10/02/2015

Apresentação do Projeto:

Será empregada a abordagem compreensiva que abarca o estudo das relações, representações, percepções, crenças e opiniões (MINAYO, 2010)
privilegiando a perspectiva das pessoas e famílias em diferentes situações de vida e cuidado. Tal abordagem nos permitirá maior aproximação com
o vivido pelas famílias apreendendo, assim, aspectos relevantes de seu cotidiano; e, também, melhor compreender como elas serão afetadas por
algumas intervenções que serão propostas no projeto. Farão parte do estudo, pessoas e suas famílias residentes no Estado de Mato Grosso e/ou
Rondônia que utilizem serviços públicos de saúde, podendo ser participantes os diferentes membros familiares, incluindo crianças, adolescentes,
adultos e idosos, desde que aceitem participar do estudo e, no caso de menores de dezoito anos ou dependentes, que assintam nesta participação
junto com seus responsáveis.

Objetivo da Pesquisa:

Compreender os potenciais de famílias em situações de vulnerabilidade que subsidiem a modelagem do cuidado

Endereço: Rua Fernado Correa da Costa nº 2367
Bairro: Boa Esperança **CEP:** 78.060-900
UF: MT **Município:** CUIABA
Telefone: (63)3615-8254 **E-mail:** shirleyfp@bol.com.br

Avaliação dos Riscos e Benefícios:

Riscos: Quanto a possíveis riscos na condução do estudo, salienta-se que a participação de pessoas e famílias na pesquisa não oferecerá qualquer risco ou
dano à sua saúde, sendo que as mesmas terão apenas o desconforto de participar da entrevista, podendo se retirar a qualquer momento.

Benefícios: Benefícios: salienta-se o compromisso em informar aos participantes da relevância dos resultados do
estudo para a formação profissional, no sentido de produzir mudanças substantivas na atuação de profissionais que lidam com pessoas e famílias nos diversos espaços assistenciais. Além disso, acreditamos que tal estudo também acarreta ganhos subjetivos aos participantes no que tange a escuta terapêutica e a relação de cuidado que é construída ao longo dos encontros.

Comentários e Considerações sobre a Pesquisa:

Pesquisa de relevância para área

Considerações sobre os Termos de apresentação obrigatória:

Folha de Rosto: adequada.

TCLE: adequado

Cronograma: adequado

Conclusões ou Pendências e Lista de Inadequações:

O pesquisador atendeu as recomendações anteriores.

Situação do Parecer:

Aprovado

Necessita Apreciação da CONEP:

Não

Considerações Finais a critério do CEP:

Projeto aprovado pelo CEP.

CUIABA, 11 de Fevereiro de 2015

Assinado por:
SHIRLEY FERREIRA PEREIRA
(Coordenador)

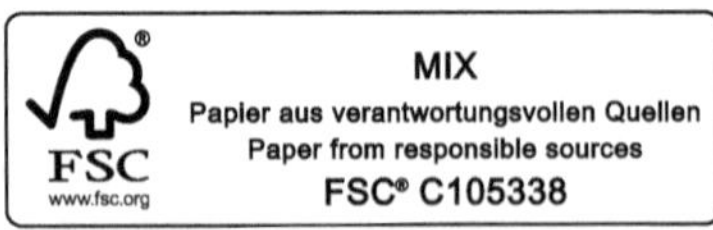

Printed by Books on Demand GmbH, Norderstedt / Germany